101 Cases

For Study

in

Pilates Teacher Training

Virginia S. Cowen, PhD

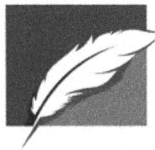

Pennate Press

ISBN 978-1-953891-19-8

Cataloging-in-Publication Data

Cowen, Virginia S., author
101 Cases for study in Pilates teacher training / Virginia S. Cowen
ISBN 978-1-953891-19-8

Library of Congress Control Number: 2020920870

All cases in this book are fictional. Any resemblance or similarity to a real person, living or dead, is coincidental and not intended by the author.

First printing November 2020

Published by
Pennate Press
An imprint of IngeniousWellness
P.O. Box 83
Piermont, NY 10968
www.pennatepress.com

Preface

I started teaching Pilates at a resort hotel with a lovely spa. Tourism and conventions brought guest from all over the world. Some were trying Pilates for the very first time, others were regular participants at a studio or gym. Pre-session screening had to be extremely efficient. The diversity in the guest population required me to think on my feet and watch very closely. The same mat class might have a guest with degenerative disc disease, one who was pregnant, a guest who had just mastered Jack Knife at her home studio, and another guest who was completely puzzled about The Hundred. I needed my critical thinking skills every day.

Pilates teachers come from a wide range of backgrounds. Regardless of whether Pilates teachers come from physical therapy, exercise physiology, dance, or business, what everyone has in common is The Pilates Method. Critical thinking skills are needed for assessment, teaching strategies, and to design Pilates exercise programs to meet the needs of a diverse array of clients. Case-based learning provides a safe space for students in Pilates teacher training programs to practice critical thinking. As an educator, I am fond of case-based learning because it is interactive.

Versions of this book were written for other fitness and wellness professions. This book was adapted for Pilates. I hope that instructors and in Pilates teacher training programs will find these narratives useful to explore ideas about communication and teaching strategies.

Virginia S. Cowen, PhD

Contents

CONTENTS

Introduction

Case-based learning provides students with the opportunity to apply critical thinking skills at all levels of education. Cases can be used to walk students through inductive reasoning needed to recognize information relevant to signs, symptoms, or disorders. Case-based learning can also be used to help students acquire deductive reasoning skills needed to develop treatment plans. Whether students are at a novice, intermediate, or advanced level, case-based learning provides context.

Whereas in medicine a case study is a presentation of a rare or unusual patient, in education a case study is a story or scenario that is used as a teaching tool. In teaching and learning, case scenarios are sometimes written in an ideal manner to present typical signs, symptoms, and progress of a disease or disorder. This does lead students through a thought process. But in practice a client's presentation is rarely ideal and often not typical.

In this book, each case is written in a realistic manner using a biopsychosocial approach. Often in case-based learning, students can fall into a "find the diagnosis" trap. For students in Pilates teacher training, it is essential to avoid this trap and instead focus information needed to make clinical decisions regarding safety and efficacy of massage treatment. An adequate amount of information is provided in each case to use it as a teaching opportunity. The cases were structured to be scientifically accurate and realistic to help guide students in the critical thinking process. Just like a real client, students will need to explore aspects of the case and make inferences to guide their search for additional information and design exercise programs.

The cases are entirely fictional but draw upon details from realistic situations. The cases were prepared to reflect demographics of the adult population in the United States and characteristics of fitness participants. The cases are 56% female, 42% male, and 2% transgender. The average age is 44. Distribution of race and occupation across the cases was designed to be slightly more diverse than the U.S. population. This was intended to encourage student learning about diversity while presenting generally accurate demographics. Due to geographical differences, the book as a whole may not be typical of Pilates clients in a specific area. Regardless of whether the cases are more or less diverse, each presents a learning opportunity.

Students sometimes become fascinated with rare and unusual disorders while ignoring common problems they will likely encounter in their future work. To help students focus on highly-prevalent diseases and disorders, cancer, hypertension, high cholesterol, diabetes, and heart disease are included in cases and in references to family members to indicate potential genetic predisposition. Even though these types of conditions are not directly treated with Pilates, students should be familiar with signs, symptoms, and diagnoses since they are likely to encounter them in practice.

Many sources for case studies use a clinical outline rather than a narrative. While using an outline details essential information for learning purposes, it does not provide a realistic scenario related to future work. The clinical outline can be confusing for Pilates teachers who do not come from a clinical background. Narratives are used in this book to reflect real-world practice. Each is written in a conversational style. The tone is a combination of lay language and clinical terminology to mirror the way clients often speak of signs, symptoms, diagnosed medical conditions, and treatments. The narrative format presents the opportunity for instructors to use this book in conjunction with health history forms, assessment tools, and research-based assignments.

Case Format

The format for each case scenario has six features:

Name. Each case is given a first name. The name contributes to each case's identity. Using a name instead of initials or an anonymous approach encourages the student to appreciate that a case represents a person. The names are fictional.

Age. Risk for some diseases and disorders rises as a person ages. The onset for other diseases and disorders occurs at a younger age. Some people look older or younger than their biological age. Others refuse to divulge their age. For teaching and learning purposes, students should be comfortable recognizing the relationship between age and health risk.

Sex. A person's sex is related to biological risk for diseases and disorders. This applies not only to hormones and the reproductive organs, but also to other conditions like heart disease and types of cancer. Sex is not the same as gender. Gender is a social identity that is associated with behaviors as well as mental and emotional health risks. Sex is included in the details for each case. Transgender cases are included to be inclusive, to reflect characteristics of the U.S. population, and to introduce health concerns for transgender persons. For teaching and learning purposes, instructors could broaden the discussion to include gender, especially when cases are used to practice client interviewing.

Race. NIH categories for race are used in this book: American Indian, Alaska Native, Asian, Black, Pacific Islander, and White. Multiracial is used as a term for cases that identify as more than one race. Race is not the same as ethnicity or culture. A person's race is related to biological risk for diseases and disorders. Culture and ethnicity influence beliefs, behaviors, and social norms. For teaching and learning purposes, instructors could broaden the discussion about a case to include culture and ethnicity.

Occupation. Occupation is included for every case. Most adults spend approximately one-third of their time at work or doing work. The tasks and the environment related to a person's occupation can increase health-related risks including (but not limited to) accidents, repetitive stress injuries, and exposure to pathogens. Sedentary occupations have higher risk for heart disease, diabetes, and other disorders linked to physical inactivity. Individuals in high-stress occupations have physical and mental health risks that may be attenuated through stress management.

Narrative. Each case includes a narrative that provides part of the case's story. The detail provided in each narrative differs depending upon the characteristics of the case and may include hobbies, lifestyle, social support, and stress management in addition to comorbid conditions, history of injury, and/or medical treatment. Family history is provided for a selection of the cases to help students recognize the impact of genetics on health and disease.

Instructors can use this space to record important information for teaching. Students can use this space for reference notes.

Learning Objectives

This book has an overarching objective to provide opportunities for students to apply concepts from Pilates to realistic case studies. Working with the case studies in this book will provide students with opportunities to:

- Appreciate the range of biological, psycho-emotional, social, and cultural factors that influence a client's well-being.

- Gain an understanding of the prevalence of common and chronic diseases/disorders.

- Recognize how to filter information in order to identify what is important in exercise program design.

- Develop clinical-thinking skills by practicing assessment, session design, and reassessment.

The format is consistent for all 101 cases, but not identical. The cases were designed as narratives with no correct answer to encourage exploration. The information provided is specific to each case. Every single detail may not be relevant depending upon how the case is used in teaching. When a client tells their story, all of the details may not be important for exercise program design. Learning how to listen to clients can help students get to know them and identify what information is essential. Working with cases provides an opportunity to practice communication skills and critical thinking.

Teaching and Learning With Cases

Using pre-written case studies for teaching has advantages. Instructors who try to provide examples from real clients may inadvertently compromise privacy and confidentiality. This is especially true when a client has an unusual presentation or the surrounding community is small. The intentional diversity in the design of these case narratives might be more diverse than the community surrounding where the program is based. This can broaden perspective for students and better prepare them with skills to serve a more diverse population.

Critical Thinking

As a teaching tool, cases connect theory to practice by providing a framework for students to apply concepts, explore possibilities, and envision potential outcomes. Case-based learning provides a safe environment for to learn to recognize risk factors and how that impacts exercise participation.

A case can be introduced to set the stage for material that will be covered including assessments. The case can then be revisited later on once material has been introduced to give students an opportunity to review and apply concepts.

In a live class session or using a discussion board in an online class, the instructor can use a dialogue to ask students thought provoking questions about the case as if the case was a real client. The aim in this method is to encourage collective thinking and problem solving through the dialogue.

Collaborative Learning

Cases can be used for collaborative activities in small groups. Students can review cases to identify and extract relevant information. This could involve underlining keywords or filling out a health history form from the perspective of the case. Students can brainstorm assessments that might reveal more information or be used to gauge effects of Pilates as a pre- and post-test.

Pairs of students can use role play to practice interview skills. One student could act as the case and the other student the Pilates teacher. Students could also complete a health history form based upon what they know about the case to identify potential questions.

Information Literacy

Pilates offers benefits to people with different health needs and movement abilities. Cases can be used to promote health information literacy to help students in teacher training gain a broader perspective about issues related to a case. Students could be asked to identify potentially relevant resource material that could be used to provide insight into the case. Students could select different cases and then share what they learned with each other.

Session Design

Cases can be used to practice designing group classes or private sessions. Students could be asked to design a small group class using several cases as participants and include recommended modifications, props, or precautions. They could also design a progressive program for an individual client that outlines sessions for several weeks—and includes plans for assessments.

Active Learning

Case-based learning provides many opportunities for discussion and interactive assignments. It adapts well to face-to-face classes, small group activities, and asynchronous distance learning. The next few pages provides an example of a template that students could use to work with a case scenario for self-directed learning.

Case Review Template

Potential Assessments

Duration and Frequency of Sessions

Exercise Progression Plan

Timeline and Plan for Reassessment

Session Ideas

Mat Exercises

Apparatus and Exercises

Props

Precautions or Modifications

101 Cases

Sarah

Age: 52

Sex: Female

Race: White

Occupation: Office Manager

Sarah has suffered from hip pain for the past few months. She describes it as an ache that she feels during movement, but does not notice when she is sitting still. She tries to stretch and use a heating pad. Sometimes she takes an over-the-counter pain reliever.

Sarah wants to take a few sessions to focus on her hip pain.

Sarah is a former professional dancer. She retired from dancing when she was 40 and currently works full time in a medical office as an office manager. During her 25-year career as a dancer she performed with a dance company and in many musical theater productions. Sarah also took daily class in different dance styles.

To offset her sedentary office job, Sarah still tries to go to dance class twice per week and take at least 10,000 steps every day.

During her dance career, Sarah suffered from injuries that she describes as "the ones that most dancers have to deal with," including a condition she describes as "snapping hip syndrome."

When Sarah was in her twenties, she was diagnosed with osteopenia. She takes dietary supplements to promote bone health, low dose aspirin, and follows a healthy diet.

Sarah's hip pain does not bother her at work. Sometimes, it flares up doing daily activities, like when she is carrying laundry up the stairs. Pain during dance class has worsened lately. She would rather modify choreography than miss class. Sarah always feels at home with other dancers.

Sarah hopes that a series of Reformer sessions might help manage her hip pain so she does not have to miss dance class.

Case Notes

Laurie

Age: 78

Sex: Female

Race: Black

Occupation: Retired administrator

Laurie has bilateral foot pain from diabetic neuropathy. She feels burning, tingling, and sometimes sharp pain. Usually it is in her feet. But sometimes it gets bad and creeps from her feet up her lower legs. Laurie tries elevating her legs, massaging her feet, and uses topical creams to ease the symptoms. These efforts provide some relief, but she has not found a recipe that works every time.

She was diagnosed with diabetes at age 11. Her symptoms came on very suddenly and she missed almost a month of 6th grade. One of Laurie's aunts died when she was very young, probably of diabetes.

Laurie credits her mother and grandmother with helping her learn to manage diabetes. She tests her blood sugar multiple times each day and gives herself insulin injections. Laurie is very careful about what she eats and scheduling her meals so she does not develop hypoglycemia. She learned to carefully monitor every cut, scrape, and wound because they took a long time to heal. When Laurie was in her late forties, she started checking her feet for wounds every night before bed.

Before she retired, she kept a footstool under her desk at work so she could elevate her feet. As the neuropathy worsened over the years, Laurie found it more difficult to take long walks. She loved walking to keep fit and relieve stress. She and her husband still take shorter walks when she can.

Laurie wants to sign up for a series of group classes focusing on her feet to help with circulation and pain relief. She is interested in trying Pilates because she heard it is gentle exercise that helps with posture. Laurie hopes she will be able to keep up in the class.

Case Notes

Felix

Age: 68

Sex: Male

Race: White

Occupation: Marketing Executive

Felix is a committed recreational athlete. He runs, cycles, and swims year-round and competes in local races. He has completed several Ironman Triathlons and marathons. His favorite event is a half marathon. Felix maintains a general training program to stay fit. He varies his regimen depending upon upcoming race schedules.

Felix has tried a lot of different exercise modalities over the years. Usually something can help alleviate aches and discomfort that can happen with intense training.

As a former high school athlete, Felix always found training fun and good for stress relief. He often participates in weekly training runs hosted by a sporting goods store and is a member of a masters swimming club. He likes getting training tips, but especially enjoys the camaraderie.

Over the years, Felix has had several minor injuries: hamstring strain, hip pain, low back pain that were easily managed with stretching, heat, ice, and rest. About 20 years ago, he had a cycling accident and separated his right shoulder. His injury was severe and left him with a deformity. He was diligent about rehabilitation exercises. He has good strength and range of motion, despite having a pronounced bump where his shoulder does not properly align.

Getting up early to train helps Felix get his mindset for the day. He likes his job and is not ready to retire. His workday can be long and sometimes his back hurts. He alternates between a sitting and standing desk and takes stretch breaks. When soreness and discomfort become problematic, he takes ibuprofen.

Felix has been feeling a little stiff and wants to loosen up.

Case Notes

Solange

Age: 42

Sex: Female

Race: White

Occupation: Paralegal

Solange has traveled extensively and been to spas all over the world. A massage at a Japanese onsen was very intense. A hair pulling session in Hong Kong was strangely relaxing. She has done gyrotonics and inverted yoga. She has meditated in the most beautiful settings. Solange also enjoys spa treatments, especially when menus offer something creative. She has tried chocolate, seaweed, coconut, and hibiscus flowers for wraps, scrubs, and feet. The possibilities seem endless. Solange has loved sampling different spa treatments; she loves how they make her skin feel.

Solange thinks adding a small group Pilates class to her wellness routine might be a nice luxury.

As a paralegal, Solange's job requires heavy concentration and high attention to detail. She has worked at the same law office for a long time. It is a small firm and they are a close group. Her work is sedentary; she sits all day.

Solange has a gym membership and tries to attend a group fitness class two or three times per week. Usually one of the dance aerobics classes fits her schedule. For Solange, the music makes the class fun and not feel like work.

A few years ago, Solange's blood pressure was elevated for the first time at her annual physical. Since then, she has taken a low dose aspirin and a fish oil supplement daily. Solange is a little overweight and tries to watch what she eats. She has a weakness for sweets.

Solange does not want to sweat. Group fitness classes are for sweating. She is looking to do something different that has more of a mind and body focus. She wants to find a class she can take on a regular basis.

Case Notes

Maury

Age: 53

Sex: Male

Race: White

Occupation: Commercial Driver

Maury has driven 18-wheelers for over 20 years. Being a commercial driver can be stressful in bad weather, or when traffic is heavy, but Maury has learned to take that in stride. He enjoys the camaraderie of other drivers and people he meets while making deliveries. No two days are ever the same.

Many of Maury's fellow drivers struggle with heart disease and diabetes. Maury wants to avoid that fate. Maury works hard to watch what he eats. He does not have much time to exercise when he is on the road. When he is home, Maury enjoys tossing a ball around with his son and taking the family dog for long hikes.

A long time ago, Maury developed pain in his right hip and low back. He was diagnosed with sciatica and went through physical therapy. Maury was diligent about doing his home exercises and kept doing them for several years. Recently, he started having hip pain again.

Maury takes a multivitamin, a garlic supplement, and vitamin C every day. His blood pressure is normal. Maury's parents are both healthy. His older brother died of a heart attack at age 49.

The current pain in Maury's hip makes it hard to get moving in the morning. When he gets out of the truck to take a break, the first few steps are difficult. Stretching helps a little.

Maury heard that Pilates is good for back pain. He wonders if it could help his hip problem. He has never taken Pilates. He wants to try a session and see if he can also learn some exercises to do when he is on the road.

Case Notes

Pablo

Age: 33

Sex: Male

Race: White

Occupation: Designer

Pablo designs custom kitchens. He loves the creative process and has built a large portfolio that highlights his work. Pablo works for a small company as part of their residential interior design staff. He spends most of his time drafting and revising plans. Pablo works with the sales department and works with carpenters, plumbers, and electricians on creative design ideas. He enjoys consultations with clients. He sketches designs by hand for initial ideas and then builds the plan on the computer.

Lately Pablo's neck and shoulders have been stiff and achy. He notices that it gets worse when he spends more time drafting designs in the office. He tries to take stretch breaks which only help temporarily. He takes an over-the-counter analgesic when he is at work. His wife tried massaging his back, but it did not feel very good.

Pablo wonders if a some private Pilates sessions might be helpful.

Pablo has been feeling irritable at work when his neck and shoulders ache. His colleagues can tell when he does not feel well by changes in his posture and the expression on his face.

Other than the neck and shoulder problem, Pablo is healthy. He jogs after work and plays in a weekend soccer league. His parents and one of his older brothers have diabetes. Pablo's other brother has had asthma since he was a child.

Pablo scheduled an introduction session to focus on his neck and shoulders. He hopes to break the discomfort and improve his posture.

Case Notes

Marilyn

Age: 27

Sex: Female

Race: White

Occupation: Business Analyst

Marilyn believes in working hard and playing hard. From high school through college, she competed in track—distance events were her specialty. She enjoyed being part of the team and made enduring friendships. Marilyn still runs 20-30 miles per week. For her it is as much a habit as it is a way to stay fit and manage stress.

When Marilyn was running in high school, she struggled with tight hamstrings. A combination of a warm-up routine, stretching, and massage helped her work through the discomfort so she could keep running. Lately her right leg has been bothering her.

Marilyn wants to take some group Reformer sessions to try to loosen up her hamstrings so she can minimize her injury risk and keep running.

Marilyn's work involves sitting at a computer or sitting in meetings. When a big project is in progress, she can end up working for 10 or 12 hours a day. This can be stressful, but Marilyn's job pays her very well and the company provides meals on long workdays. It can be difficult to schedule running time when she is involved in a big project.

Marilyn's father died from mesothelioma when he was 48. Her mother struggled with some depression at that time. Marilyn is close to her brothers and sisters. They rallied around their mother and she is doing better.

Marilyn has never suffered from any major injuries. She has low blood pressure. She gets an annual physical, has regular dental checkups, and sees a dermatologist to cope with sensitive skin.

Updating her hamstring care routine is Marilyn's current goal so she can stick to her running routine.

Case Notes

Delilah

Age: 25

Sex: Female

Race: White

Occupation: Waitress

Delilah is a full-time waitress and a part-time actress. She moved to the city after graduating from college and is working hard to launch her acting career. Delilah's work schedule at the restaurant varies weekly. She can switch shifts with other waitstaff to take auditions and go to rehearsals. While nearly all of Delilah's time involves waitressing or acting, she wants to do everything she can to launch her acting career.

A few weeks ago, Delilah landed a small role in a workshop production of a new play. She was excited to begin rehearsals. Unfortunately, the role does not pay very much so she must continue working at the restaurant. Her neck and shoulders are tense and sore. Delilah feels very tired at the end of her restaurant shifts. Between rehearsals, studying her part, and waitressing, she is getting run-down. She is too tired to go running or to the gym.

When Delilah was in high school, she was in a car crash. Delilah was a passenger in the front seat and her friend was driving. Delilah and her friend both sustained whiplash injuries. Delilah spent weeks wearing a neck brace and taking medication. She then received a few months of treatment from a chiropractor. Recovery was slow. She continued to have headaches and occasional pain in her jaw. Other than that, she is healthy.

Delilah's mother is a breast cancer survivor. Her father takes medication for hypertension. Delilah has one sister who suffers from debilitating migraine headaches.

Delilah's neck and shoulder tension makes waitressing difficult. Her friend suggested that Pilates might improve her posture and manage the discomfort so she can get through her restaurant shifts.

Case Notes

Shmuel

Age: 47

Sex: Male

Race: White

Occupation: Musician

Shmuel is a professional violinist. He makes a living teaching private lessons, playing chamber music, and as a substitute in different orchestras. He started playing when he was very young. Shmuel plays every day either at rehearsals, in a performance, or practicing. When Shmuel practices, it is for about two hours straight. It can be intense if he is learning a new work or trying to master a difficult passage. Even when it is difficult, Shmuel loves playing the violin.

About a year ago, Shmuel started having back pain. It is usually an intermittent dull ache. Occasionally he feels a sharper pain when he stands up after sitting for a long time. This is very awkward when it happens at the end of a performance; he tries not to grimace when the audience can see him. Shmuel needs to find a way to manage this back pain.

Shmuel does not exercise, but he does walk a lot. Usually he is carrying a briefcase and his violin and rushing from a rehearsal to teach a lesson. Over the years he has slowly gained weight. His blood pressure and cholesterol are a little high, but still in the normal range. He takes low dose aspirin and a multivitamin every day. Shmuel tries to eat a healthy diet and manages to do so about half the time. Late-night dinners after a performance can be challenging to manage.

Shmuel's older brother had a myocardial infarction a few years ago. He completed cardiac rehabilitation and is doing well. Their father died from heart disease complications when he was 62. Their mother died a year later after a long battle with emphysema. Playing the violin helped Shmuel cope with the loss of his parents. For him, playing is as much about stress management as making music.

The back pain is getting in the way of Shmuel's life and livelihood. He read an article about Pilates and wants to give it a try.

Case Notes

Seamus

Age: 32

Sex: Male

Race: White

Occupation: Carpenter

Seamus has been interested in carpentry since he was a little boy. His grandfather built custom cabinetry and Seamus loved to visit his workshop. Seamus entered a training program after he graduated high school, completed an apprenticeship and started working in commercial construction. For fun, Seamus also designs and builds custom furniture.

Seamus has always had trouble with his left knee. When he was young, he sustained a meniscus tear while playing soccer. Pain flares up occasionally, and sometimes his left leg feels weak. His work involves physical labor. When he is uncomfortable, pain relievers help him get through the day.

A few years ago, Seamus joined a friend doing a high-intensity interval training program. Except for vacations and holidays, they consistently train together three or four days per week. They enjoy the competitive nature of the program. Seamus credits the program with helping him stay fit, managing his weight, and keeping his blood pressure in check. The exercise program and his hobby building furniture are stress management for Seamus.

His father, who was diagnosed with hypertension in his forties, takes medication, and has to watch what he eats. His mother and his two younger sisters struggle with their weight. Seamus knows that he needs to stay fit in order to keep up with the demands of his job.

When his knee problem flares up it makes Seamus anxious. He still tries to workout but has to modify some of the exercises and ice his knee when they finish. Seamus is looking to add something to his routine to help his knee pain.

Case Notes

Jane

Age: 53

Sex: Female

Race: White

Occupation: Casting Director

In her job as a casting director, Jane does a lot of collaboration. When she is starting a new project, there are lots of meetings with producers, directors, and actors. That makes for very long days. Afterwards, she and her assistant go through hundreds of submissions to find the right actors for the job. For Jane, each job is an intricate puzzle that feels like a binge. She loves it.

Jane is healthy for her age, although she is a bit overweight. She exercises daily (stationary cycling, Pilates, or yoga.) Jane was an athlete growing up. For her, playing softball and basketball was as much about getting fit as the chance to compete. She credits her competitive nature to her professional success. Her daily exercise session is very important to her to keep moving and manage stress.

Jane tries to eat a balanced diet which is difficult with all of the lunch and dinner meetings she must attend. At her last annual physical, her blood pressure was at the high end of the normal range.

Two years ago, Jane had cataract surgery. It was the first—and only—time she had any type of surgery other than wisdom teeth removal when she was a teen. Her mother (a nonsmoker) died from lung cancer at age 68. Jane's father is a healthy 83-year-old who stays active volunteering. Her older brother is a little overweight and he takes daily medication for hypertension.

Jane booked a spa day for a mini vacation. She plans to start the day a private Pilates session and follow that with a massage and facial. She wants to relax and take a break before her next big project begins.

Case Notes

Otto

Age: 47

Sex: Male

Race: Multiracial

Occupation: Hair Stylist

Otto has known since he was a little boy that he wanted to work with hair. He got in trouble when he was seven for cutting the hair on his sister's dolls. Otto started taking cosmetology classes when he was in high school and worked weekends at an upscale salon as an assistant. As soon as he got his license, Otto started working as a stylist. He loves the creative process for each cut, color, or style. Otto has built a following of devoted clients. His schedule is packed from open to close. Lately, Otto has been feeling unusually run-down.

Otto does not really exercise. He walks his dog twice a day and is on his feet all day in the salon. A few weeks ago, when Otto and his girlfriend were walking their dog in the park, Otto started to feel dizzy and out of breath. They took a break to sit on a bench, and after that Otto felt better.

Otto is very slender. For his entire life, no matter what he ate, he has never been able to put on weight. His blood pressure has always been on the low end of normal. He is rarely sick and does not currently take any medications. Otto is fastidious about his oral health; he gets his teeth cleaned on a regular schedule. His father needed dentures in his late forties. Otto wants to avoid that fate. Otto's mother has taken medication for thyroid disease for many years.

Usually when Otto gets run-down, he tries to relax, read, and spend time with his girlfriend and dog. He knows that he should try to do some sort of exercise to break his cycle of fatigue. He does not like to sweat. His girlfriend suggested that he try Pilates to help his posture and his overall fitness.

Case Notes

Barbara

Age: 61

Sex: Female

Race: Black

Occupation: Nonprofit Executive

Barbara is the executive director of a nonprofit organization that matches older adults with employment opportunities. Although her job can be stressful, she finds her work very fulfilling. Barbara has worked in the nonprofit sector for her entire career. She was recruited for her current job based upon her work in community engagement programs. Barbara loves connecting with and serving members of the community.

Barbara's feet are bothering her again. Since she was in her forties, Barbara has suffered from neuropathy in her feet and lower legs. She underwent many diagnostic tests that were all inconclusive. She does not have diabetes. She has never taken any medications that are known to increase risk, nor has she suffered any injury to her legs or feet. When the problem began, Barbara started wearing custom orthotics. When she can take her shoes off at work, she rolls her foot on a golf ball. Barbara elevates her feet at night and uses a topical analgesic before bed that provides some relief.

Barbara feet often cramp and tingle. They easily get swollen when she stands for long periods of time. Although loss of sensation is characteristic of neuropathy, Barbara does not have numbness. Her podiatrist finds that unusual.

Two of Barbara's sisters are overweight and have Type 2 diabetes. Neither has diabetic neuropathy or foot pain. Their mother died at age 78 after suffering a stroke. Barbara never met her father, so she knows very little about his health history.

Barbara hopes that exercise that does not require her to stand will help her get fit and provide relief from her foot problems.

Case Notes

Jerry

Age: 38

Sex: Male

Race: White

Occupation: Bank Officer

Jerry has had persistent lower-back discomfort for years. It is a combination of soreness and stiffness. Occasionally it gets worse and Jerry feels achy. When he tries to stretch, his low back feels weak. Sometimes the discomfort makes it difficult to concentrate at work. When that happens, he uses an over-the-counter analgesic.

Despite being active, Jerry has been overweight all of his life. He played football and baseball when he was growing up. He did not like conditioning but enjoyed games and scrimmage. Jerry and his husband met in a hiking club and share a love of horseback riding. They try to go hiking or riding every weekend. They gave up their gym memberships a long time ago since neither of them enjoyed lifting weights.

Over the years, Jerry has tried physical therapy, acupuncture, and several months of spinal manipulations by a chiropractor. These provided relief in the short term, but the low back discomfort eventually came back. His physical therapist suggested that being overweight might contribute to the problem. Despite trying dozens of diets, Jerry has never been able to lose weight.

Jerry was 16 when his father died in an accident. His mother struggled with depression, but medication and therapy helped her recover. She remarried and Jerry has a cordial relationship with his stepfather. Jerry knows little about his father's health history, but his paternal grandfather is 86 and plays golf several times a week. Jerry's paternal grandmother died of cancer at age 77.

Jerry is on a mission to find something to help his back feel better. He wants to find a better solution than medication. Jerry hopes Pilates might help.

Case Notes

Irving

Age: 41

Sex: Male

Race: Asian

Occupation: Radiologist

Irving's shoulder has been bothering him again. About eight or nine years ago, he sustained a torn rotator cuff while using the overhead press machine at the gym. He remembers it like it happened yesterday. In the middle of his second set he felt a pop and then a searing pain in his right shoulder. He was diagnosed with a rotator cuff tear and his orthopedist advised a conservative treatment approach. After a few weeks of physical therapy, Irving was able to regain most of his shoulder's range of motion without discomfort. It took a long time for the pain to go away completely.

After his original shoulder injury, Irving stopped lifting weights. Not long ago, the pain came back. Irving does not remember doing anything specific this time. but he felt the same pain from the old injury when he put his arm over his head to pull on a t-shirt. He knows that old injuries have a way of flaring up.

Irving remembers working on stretches for his posture during physical therapy. He wonders if Pilates have a similar benefit.

Irving's work involves long days staring at computer screen reading images. Every so often at work, he feels a twinge in his right shoulder when he moves the computer mouse a certain way. If he rubs his shoulder the pain goes away.

Irving has a normal body weight, tries to eat a balanced diet, and takes daily medication for hypertension. Other than that, he is healthy. Irving's father was recently diagnosed with atherosclerosis and prescribed medication. Irving's mother has modified their diet and makes sure they take daily walks.

Irving wants to try Pilates to see if it can help the pain in his shoulder.

Case Notes

Martina

Age: 34

Sex: Female

Race: White

Occupation: Electrician

Martina works on large commercial construction projects. Her work as a union electrician takes her to different sites all over the city. Sometimes when she installs wiring or fixtures, she works very small and tight spaces. This can require her to bend and twist into awkward positions. Her back and neck can get sore very quickly. Despite the occasional discomfort, Martina likes her work. It pays well, has good benefits, and there is a lot of variety to her work.

Martina stretches to alleviate soreness in her neck and back. She wonders if core strengthening could help.

Three or four times per week, Martina works out on the cardio equipment at the gym and enjoys taking one of the dance classes. Despite being active, she is a little bit overweight. Martina lives with her mother who loves to cook—not always the healthiest dishes. Martina enjoys going out for drinks with her friends. She admits that her eating habits could be better.

Martina's parents separated when she was young. She and her younger sister visit their father regularly and remain close to him. Her mother takes a daily medication to manage her asthma. Martina's younger sister also has asthma. A few years ago, her father had a mild heart attack. He went through cardiac rehabilitation, started exercising, and changed his diet.

Martina's back and neck problems are not related to a workplace injury, so treatment is not covered by worker's compensation. She is trying to find a way to manage it on her own.

Martina is curious to see whether a series of Pilates classes could help her neck and back to alleviate the discomfort.

Case Notes

Amanda

Age: 47

Sex: Female

Race: Multiracial

Occupation: Entrepreneur

After enjoying a successful corporate career, Amanda launched her own soap and fragrance company. She manufactures and sells unique scents and is carving out a niche in the luxury gift market. Her products are sold in spas, boutiques, and gift shops all across the country. Amanda works long days contacting suppliers, supervising formulators, and making sales calls. It is exhausting and rewarding.

Amanda sustained an ankle sprain about a year ago. She was rushing to make a flight and twisted her left ankle. She managed to make it through that trip by applying ice every chance she got. An X-ray was negative—no bones were broken or dislocated. Her ankle still seems weak, so she feels that it did not heal properly. Amanda loves wearing high-heeled shoes and is annoyed that her ankle is not back to normal.

Amanda's brother raves about Pilates. He is urging her to try a few sessions.

Amanda takes medication for hypertension. She is prediabetic, so she must be careful about her diet. She has been overweight since she was a child. Her mother has diabetes and her father has heart disease. Both take medication. Since diagnosis, they have been trying to eat healthier, but they admit that is difficult.

Amanda's older brother is a former professional athlete who still works out every day.

Amanda hopes that Pilates could help her stay fit and straighten out whatever is still going wrong in her ankle. She is willing to try anything to be able to wear heels with confidence.

Case Notes

Saachi

Age: 42

Sex: Female

Race: Asian

Occupation: Dentist

Saachi recently recovered from malaria. Six months ago, she traveled to India for a family wedding. A few days after she returned home, she developed mild flu-like symptoms (headache, fever, and chills). The symptoms were intermittent, but persistent. Malaria is common in the area she visited. Based upon Saachi's travel history, her primary care provider referred her to an infectious disease specialist. Saachi was diagnosed with malaria. She took leave from work, completed a course of medication, and eventually began to feel better.

Saachi has had a hard time regaining energy. She wants to try something new to help her feel recharged and refreshed.

Saachi has been trying to walk every morning to build stamina and get her energy back. She has been a vegetarian all of her life. She had gestational diabetes when she was pregnant with her second child. She knows that increases her risk for Type 2 Diabetes, so she tries to pay careful attention to her diet. Both of her parents both developed Type 2 diabetes in their fifties, but her older brother does not have diabetes.

Saachi has occasional back pain when she is at work. It is relatively mild. If she stretches, the discomfort usually goes away.

Saachi is looking for low intensity exercise. She has no interest in trying to exert or push herself. Saachi wants to put lingering feelings of fatigue from malaria behind her.

Case Notes

Eddie

Age: 36

Sex: Male

Race: White

Occupation: Plumber

Eddie followed his father into the plumbing and heating industry. His father heads the company and his mother handles the administrative tasks. Eddie loves the technical aspects of his work. Together they have built a successful family business. Eddie enjoys working with his family because they have a good rapport. His friends have much more stressful jobs. Eddie counts himself lucky.

Eddie loves playing basketball. He played in recreational youth leagues and on his high school team. Whenever he can, Eddie plays pick-up games with his friends. Sometimes his knees hurt after playing. Usually it feels better after some ice and rest. Lately his knees hurt at the end of a workday.

Eddie's girlfriend suggested he try a Pilates mat class to improve his flexibility.

Other than the knee problems, Eddie is healthy. He has never smoked, drinks alcohol in moderation, and tries to eat a healthy diet. Eddie has very fair skin and regularly sees a dermatologist. Some of his freckles were found to be cancerous after they were surgically removed. Eddie's parents are both healthy and so are his grandparents. All four of them are still alive. Eddie's younger sister was diagnosed with preeclampsia when she was pregnant.

But her baby was born healthy and she is doing well with blood pressure now in the normal range. Eddie considers himself blessed and says he has good genes.

Eddie thinks Pilates is for women, but he is looking for something to help manage his knee discomfort. He really needs something to help him get through the workday and recover after playing basketball.

Case Notes

Rosie

Age: 55

Sex: Female

Race: White

Occupation: Banker

Rosie started experiencing facial tics a few months ago. She thinks it is related to increased stress. Work has been difficult because her company went through a merger and reorganization is ongoing. Many of her colleagues are nervous about job stability. Uncertainty is very stressful for Rosie.

When Rosie was in her early twenties, she was diagnosed with generalized anxiety disorder. She struggled to make it through college and was working at her first professional job. Rosie was worrying about work, paying her bills, and trying to make friends. Worry and stress became constant. Rosie sought help through an employee assistance program at work. She was diagnosed, started taking medication, and began working on stress management. It helped her manage her anxiety. Rosie still takes daily medication and makes time to relax and recover at the end of the day. She cuddles with her cat and watches television. That helps her de-stress after all of the uncertainty at work.

For Rosie, a private exercise session is a special treat. She wants to try Pilates.

Rosie's father died a few years ago after a long battle with prostate cancer. Her mother died of a heart attack when Rosie was very young. Rosie and her younger sister were raised by their father, and they were a very close family. The onset of the facial tic is not unusual for Rosie. She had one when she was in high school that went away during college.

Rosie knows that exercise cannot resolve the facial tic, but she hopes learning some gentle exercise can add to her stress-management activities. Maybe that will help the tic go away this time.

Case Notes

Raimondo

Age: 28

Sex: Male

Race: Black

Occupation: Retail Manager

Raimondo is tired. He is on his feet all day at work serving customers, supervising associates, and managing store operations. Raimondo says he has lots of energy while he is at work; mostly because he enjoys the customers and likes his co-workers. When he gets home in the evening, he feels drained.

Raimondo reserved a spot in a group reformer class because he is seeking an escape from feeling tired. He wonders if gentle exercise will add something fresh to his routine.

Raimondo is typically very active. He works out at the gym three or four mornings a week. One of his friends is a personal trainer, so he designed a training routine that Raimondo tries to follow. This usually includes stationary cycling, a circuit on the stacked weight machines, and some core work. When he is pressed for time, he skips the cycling so he can do the weight routine. On days that he does not go to the gym, he tries to stretch at home.

His commitment to being active is influenced by his parents. They have long struggled with weight issues and both have hypertension and Type 2 diabetes. Raimondo is trying to avoid the same problems.

Other than spraining an ankle playing basketball in high school, he has not had any injuries other than minor cuts and bruises.

Raimondo's tiredness seems to have gotten worse recently, even after a good night's sleep. Cleaning his apartment and doing laundry seem like enormous chores. In the past few months, he cancelled plans with friends a few times because he was just too tired after a long week.

Raimondo is hoping he might like Pilates enough to add it to his routine.

Case Notes

Charlotte

Age: 72

Sex: Female

Race: White

Occupation: Nonprofit Executive

Charlotte is a development officer at a performing arts facility. She manages fundraising activities, plans campaigns, and solicits new donors. Charlotte enjoys her work because it is very people-centric, and she is passionate about music, dance, and theatre.

Charlotte's neck has been bothering her for a few weeks. The problem started when she sat too close to the air conditioner during a meeting. When she woke up the morning after the meeting, Charlotte felt a sharp pain in her neck. A heat wrap and over-the-counter analgesic helped her feel a little better, but the problem has not gone away.

Charlotte needs help with her aching neck.

A lot of Charlotte's social life centers around work. She attends performances several nights a week to meet with donors and potential donors. Luncheons, dinners, and receptions are an important part of Charlotte's work. She has learned to watch what she eats and drinks so she can maintain a reasonably healthy diet. Charlotte considers herself to be hearty and healthy for her age. She enjoys playing bridge with her friends, belongs to a hiking club, and plays in an adult recreational tennis league. Charlotte takes supplements (calcium and vitamin D) and drinks peppermint tea every morning. Her blood pressure and blood sugar are normal, and she maintains a healthy body weight.

Charlotte's mother died in her early eighties of complications from emphysema. She smoked cigarettes for many years. Charlotte's father died a few years before that from pneumonia. Both of Charlotte's younger brothers take medication for hypertension.

Charlotte hopes that Pilates might help with her posture and the problem with her neck.

Case Notes

Carol

Age: 43

Sex: Female

Race: Asian

Occupation: Nurse

Carol works in the emergency department of a large regional hospital. No two shifts are ever the same. Patients with traumatic injuries, acute illness, and unexplained symptoms arrive around the clock. Sometimes it is a steady flow of new patients, other times it is a rush. Even when it is quiet, there is always something to do.

Carol's neck is often sore by the end of her shift. She has tried to figure out if it is related to something she is doing while she works, but she has never been able to link the soreness to a specific movement, an activity, or even her posture. The problem does not happen with every shift; sometimes she has no discomfort at all. When the emergency department gets busy, Carol has too many things to do to think about her neck.

Carol has read about Pilates and wonders if she could do the exercises since she has so many problems with her neck.

Carol and her husband have one daughter who is in college. Carol's father died two years ago from stomach cancer. After that, her mother moved in to live with them. Carol is thankful because she can keep tabs on her. Carol's mother likes to keep busy, so she helps with housework and cooking. This is useful, given the length of Carol's shifts on days she works.

Neither Carol nor her mother have any serious health problems. They follow a healthy diet, walk, and do crafts to relax. Her father rarely had any health problems until he was diagnosed with stomach cancer. Both of Carol's grandmothers are alive and thriving in assisted living communities.

If Pilates does not make Carol's neck problem worse, she might add it to her routine for stress management and fitness.

Case Notes

Tommie

Age: 27

Sex: Male

Race: Multiracial

Occupation: Artist

Tommie is a fine artist who makes sculptures out of fabric, metal, and wood. He started out as an assistant to a well-known artist who does installations and performance art. Tommie struck out on his own two years ago when he was able to find an affordable studio space. He entered sculptures in a few art shows and hired a social media coordinator to show his work online. He has gotten a few commissions based upon references from previous clients. Tommie's career is starting to blossom. He is excited and nervous.

For a few weeks, Tommie has had pain in both of his calves. The muscles feel tight. Sometimes his legs cramp in the middle of the night. He has to get out of bed and stretch to make the cramp go away.

Tommie thinks changing up his exercise routine might help his legs.

Tommie works hard to keep himself in good shape. He works out at a gym six days a week and watches what he eats. He drinks in moderation and enjoys salsa dancing. He dresses stylishly. He always tries to present himself well because networking is important in his work.

When Tommie was in high school, his father had a sudden onset of chest pain. He recovered fully after cardiac catheterization and a stent. Tommie's mother has Graves' disease and takes daily medication. Tommie has an older sister that suffered from postpartum depression after her second child was born.

Tommie has done a lot of different types of exercise. This will be the first time he has tried Pilates.

Case Notes

Joan

Age: 68

Sex: Female

Race: White

Occupation: Editor

Joan loves to run. She runs 25-30 miles every week by herself or with a running club. She started running at age 36 after her daughter was born. Joan wanted to try to get in shape, so she got a secondhand jogging stroller and set out with her daughter to a nearby park. Soon she met other runners, joined a running group, and a few years later began entering recreational races a few times a year. She has made many friends through running.

Joan's left hip and knee have been bothering her lately. Stretching and heat help—but only a little. A runner friend suggested she try Pilates.

Before she started running, Joan was never athletic. She did not play sports as a child and did the minimum in physical education class. She was rarely picked first for a team and never did well on fitness tests. For Joan, running makes up for that. She is now very fit for a woman her age.

Joan and her husband enjoy good food and fine wine. She can be a hearty eater thanks to all of her running. She takes a multivitamin and drinks coffee every morning. Joan stretches before and after every run.

Five years ago, Joan's parents died within a few months of each other. Her father suffered from dementia; her mother became ill with pneumonia. Joan is an only child.

Joan partially retired from her job at a publishing company. She still works part time on projects. Her boss and colleagues appreciate her expertise. She hopes to try to stay active and fit into her senior years by running, but the problems in her hip and knee are bothersome.

Joan hopes a series of group Pilates sessions will stretch out her legs and help strengthen her core muscles.

Case Notes

James

Age: 20

Sex: Male

Race: White

Occupation: Warehouse Stocker

James has a keen sense of organization. It comes in handy in his job moving boxes and materials in and out of the warehouse. He started working at the warehouse through a program that matched elite athletes with employment opportunities offering flexibility for training and competition.

James competes in archery. He first learned archery in a summer camp. He begged his parents to let him take classes at a local archery club. James showed talent and skill and was invited to join the competitive youth team. He has been an archer ever since.

His lower back has been bothering him lately. It feels stiff and weak. One of his friends suggested that he might lack adequate core strength.

James complements his training with the archery club with stretching, yoga, and meditation. James shoots or does cross training every day. He never takes a day off.

James has three younger sisters that he adores. His father takes medication for hypertension. His mother struggles with her weight. His family is very supportive of him. They travel to his tournaments whenever they can.

James is on a tight budget. He bought a package of group classes to try Pilates. He hopes it can loosen up his lower back and resolve the problem.

Case Notes

Lucy

Age: 69

Sex: Female

Race: White

Occupation: Retired Teacher

Lucy taught elementary school for 40 years. She prided herself on having an orderly classroom. Lucy enjoyed watching her students grow up knowing she played an important part in their lives. Since retiring, Lucy has kept busy volunteering for several community organizations and knitting. Lucy finds knitting to be a perfect balance of relaxation and creativity. As soon as she finishes one project, she starts another.

Lately Lucy's hands have been bothering her. She was diagnosed with osteoarthritis when she was in her early forties. Her hands and neck bother her the most. She was treated with neck traction and advised to use a topical cream for her hands. When her hands hurt, Lucy cannot knit. That is upsetting for her.

Lucy has never done Pilates. One of her friends suggested she might try it since she needs to exercise. Lucy is not sure that it will provide relief of her discomfort.

Lucy's mother had osteoarthritis in her spine. Lucy's daughter has osteoarthritis in her knees, so Lucy believes it is hereditary.

Her husband died suddenly from heart disease about ten years ago. That was a wake-up call for Lucy. She changed her eating habits and quit smoking cigarettes. Retiring from teaching was difficult. But she found a sense of purpose in her volunteer work.

The problems with her hands do not interfere with volunteering, household chores, or really anything else but knitting. If Lucy has to give up knitting, she does not know what she will do.

Lucy is not very excited about Pilates. But she is willing to try things to help her regain pain-free use of her hands so she can knit.

Case Notes

Nayla

Age: 32

Sex: Female

Race: Black

Occupation: Respiratory Therapist

Nayla is a married mother of two children. After they started school, she completed her respiratory therapy degree and obtained her license. Nayla works per diem in an academic health center. Her workdays are long, but she finds it rewarding. On days she works, Nayla's husband gets the children to school and her mother watches them after school. Nayla is grateful for the support from her family.

Recently, Nayla began having headaches. After a series of medical appointments, she was diagnosed with migraines and given medication. Thankfully, the headaches rarely happen when she is at work. But when she gets one on a day off, she knows it is a burden on her family. Nayla thinks stress is a trigger for her headaches.

Nayla's husband bought a gift certificate for a boutique fitness studio as a surprise. He hopes some exercise it might help her migraines.

Nayla developed gestational diabetes during both of her pregnancies. She worked hard to eat right and exercise after her babies were born to reduce risk of Type 2 diabetes. Her mother and father are both overweight and take medication for hypertension. Nayla's maternal grandmother has Type 2 diabetes. None of her other grandparents lived past age 65.

Nayla is worried about her migraines. She knows she should exercise and has read about Pilates. Nayla thinks that it sounds a little bit confusing, but she is interested to try.

Case Notes

Tanya

Age: 49

Sex: Female

Race: White

Occupation: Security Guard

Tanya works the security night shift at a manufacturing facility. She relishes the peace and quiet as she makes her rounds. On days that she works a shift, her fitness tracker usually tallies at least 15,000 steps. Tanya has explored every corner of the facility.

Her back often hurts at the end of her shift. It is a combination of ache and tightness. The discomfort is intermittent. Tanya cannot figure out the pattern or what makes it worse some days more than others. She has tried different work shoes and inserts, but nothing seems to help.

Tanya needs to do something about her aching back.

Tanya is a single mother of two. Her son joined the army and her daughter is in cosmetology school. She worked hard to raise them on her own. She often worked two jobs to make ends meet. Tanya is proud that they both graduated from high school and have found careers. Her son is living far away, and she misses him. Her daughter plans to move out on her own as soon as she can save enough money. Tanya has mixed feelings about living alone because she really enjoys spending time with her children.

Tanya has chronic obstructive pulmonary disease. She quit smoking ten years ago. Tanya thinks all of the walking she does at work helps her stay healthy. She cannot walk very fast because she can easily become out of breath, but it is important for her to keep going, one foot in front of the other. Just like she has all of her life.

Tanya's back seems to hurt more often these days. She knows that she needs to figure out a plan so that she can keep working. She read that Pilates is good for back pain, so she wants to join a group class.

Case Notes

Aurora

Age: 62

Sex: Female

Race: Alaska Native

Occupation: Nurse Practitioner

Aurora's right knee and hip are bothering her again. They were injured in an automobile crash when she was in high school. She hit a moose. It was a frightening accident that totaled her truck. Aurora was lucky that she was not killed. She underwent several surgeries to repair fractures to her right leg. Then she spent many months in rehabilitation and had to miss a whole semester of high school. A positive outcome of the experience was that it piqued her interest in a career in healthcare. After her children were born, Aurora started college part-time. With support from her family, she eventually finished her degrees and obtained her nurse practitioner license. She now works in a women's health clinic.

Problems with her right leg seem to flare up occasionally with no warning. Sometimes it happens at work. When she is active her right leg always feels weaker than the left. She and her husband enjoy outdoor activities like camping, hiking, and snowshoeing. She has long followed a routine of stretching, elevating and bolstering her leg, and applying heat. That helps her recover.

Aurora wonders if gentle exercises that really focuses on her leg, posture, and gait might help.

Aurora takes medication for hypertension and high cholesterol. Both of her parents died from complications related to Type 2 diabetes. Her older brother and older sister also have Type 2 diabetes. Aurora's younger sister has hypertension.

Aurora knows she is getting older and wants to be able to stay active. She has tried yoga, tai chi, and gotten massages to condition her right leg. She has never tried Pilates.

Case Notes

Ella

Age: 28

Sex: Female

Race: White

Occupation: Musician

Ella is a very busy musician. Her band's first album sold well, and they hired a new manager. They are working with their label on songs for the next album. The plan is to outline the tour while they are recording and mixing so they can time the tour with the second album's release. The whole band is excited and nervous.

Ella sings and plays guitar, clarinet, and tenor saxophone. She has been a musician for as long as she can remember. When the band got together in college, Ella felt that she had found a second family. They make music together, tease each other, and support each other. She leaned on her bandmates when her boyfriend broke up with her a few months ago.

For about a year, Ella has been having headaches and pain in her jaw. It comes and goes and is mostly on the right side. Sometimes pain seems to radiate down to her shoulder and arm. .

Ella comes from a large family. She has two brothers and three sisters. Growing up, they were very active in their church. The whole family sang in the church choir and played for services. Going away to college was difficult for Ella because she missed her family. It was a little bit easier for her to make the choice to move to the city for the band because her family supported her.

When Ella was in college, her mother had a breast cancer scare. The lump turned out to be benign. Ella's father takes a daily low dose aspirin. Her youngest sister has cerebral palsy and uses a wheelchair. Ella misses her the most because she is so sweet and funny.

Ella knows she needs to exercise. She needs to find something to do that will not exacerbate her headaches and jaw pain.

Case Notes

Walter

Age: 50

Sex: Male

Race: Black

Occupation: General Contractor

Walter cannot sleep. He has trouble falling asleep and staying asleep. He is not worrying. His mind races thinking about all sorts of things from work, to sports, to current events. He feels that his brain is so full that it is difficult to shut off when it is time for bed.

Walter does home renovations. His business is booming. He gets most of his clients from referrals. They are generally pleasant, despite the stressful nature of home renovation. It is easy when the homeowners move to a hotel while their home is being renovated, but that does not always happen. Still he likes his clients and loves his work.

Everything is good with Walter's family. His son is in college on a sports scholarship. His daughter is doing well in high school. Walter's wife is a nurse in a large medical practice. Professionally and financially, they are doing well. However, Walter cannot sleep.

One of his painters suggested Walter try a Pilates class.

Walter was a high school athlete but rarely works out these days. He is a little overweight but has no chronic health problems. Much of Walter's work is very physical: climbing ladders, twisting to connect something, carrying supplies and equipment.

Despite his age, he rarely has a problem getting things done on the job.

Walter's father takes medication for hypertension and cholesterol. He also suffers from sleep apnea. Walter's mother is prediabetic. She started watching her diet and testing her blood sugar. Walter's sister is a happy, healthy, and busy mother of three.

Walter's primary care provider offered to prescribe medication to help him sleep, but Walter wants to avoid medication. He is looking for alternative ways to help him sleep. His primary care provider told him that exercise might help.

Case Notes

Therese

Age: 46

Sex: Female

Race: White

Occupation: Investment Banker

Therese has always been an overachiever. She followed her older brothers into hockey when she was eight. All three children played on traveling teams. It required a lot of organization, but the family lived and breathed hockey. Therese's father had some flexibility in his job as a consultant. Her mother was a novelist and could take her work anywhere. Together, they made sure the children got to games, schoolwork was completed, and their house was in order.

Therese graduated near the top of her class in high school and earned an academic scholarship to university. Then she went to work in banking. It suited her competitive nature. She still plays hockey once a week in a women's recreational league.

A little over a year ago, Therese tripped and fell at work. It happened suddenly, so she did not have time to brace herself. She injured her right arm and broke her nose. She had surgery on her nose and did some physical therapy for her shoulder and arm. When she returned to work, her colleagues teased her, but it was good-natured so she took it in stride.

Every so often Therese's elbow still bothers her. A friend suggested that gentle movement could work out some stiffness.

Other than the arm issues, Therese does not have any chronic health problems. Her parents both take medication for hypertension. One of her brothers had an angioplasty. Another has chronic back pain. In general, her family is very healthy.

Therese's boyfriend gave her a spa gift certificate. She hopes that a private Pilates session could show her if regular sessions might be good for her shoulder and right arm.

Case Notes

Mike

Age: 37

Sex: Male

Race: White

Occupation: Lighting Designer

Mike is a lighting designer for the hospitality industry. He currently works at a resort, planning and installing lighting displays for meetings and conferences. In addition to making sure everything is properly illuminated for safety, he creates unique displays to showcase conference sponsors.

Early in his career, Mike hit his head on some theatre scaffolding. He got a nasty gash on his forehead and ended up with a concussion. Mike needed stitches and was required to rest. Mike started having headaches. He would have one every few months. He was diagnosed with post-concussion syndrome and was prescribed pain medication. Mike does not like taking the pain medication because it makes him drowsy.

Mike and his husband are on vacation. They scheduled a spa day and plan to start with a group Pilates mat class.

Except for the headaches, Mike is healthy. Normal blood pressure, good resting heart rate, and normal body mass index. He tries to eat well and lifts weights at the gym three times per week. He sustained a few injuries playing sports growing up, but none contributed to lingering symptoms.

Mike was adopted at birth. He has no information about his biological parents' health history. He does not know if he has hereditary risk for heart disease, diabetes, cancer, or any other conditions. That makes filling out health history forms difficult.

Mike wrote about his post-concussion syndrome on his client intake form, but he is not currently suffering from headaches. He just wants to relax and recharge.

Case Notes

Merrill

Age: 55

Sex: Transgender

Race: White

Occupation: Counselor

Merrill is a counselor at an at-risk youth center. The urban center provides services for teens and adolescents from a variety of backgrounds. Issues the youth face range from homelessness, abuse, addiction, and violence to eating disorders and self-harming behaviors. Merrill's job is individual and group counseling.

On days when Merrill's job is intense, it causes neck and shoulder aches. This is not exactly pain, just tension and discomfort.

Merrill gets regular massages and occasionally goes to yoga class. He has never tried Pilates.

Merrill was born female and began living as a man when he was in his early twenties. After graduating college and moving to a new city where he knew no one, he found work at a restaurant and made friends. He changed the way he dressed and wore his hair and created his new identity. When Merrill decided to start living as a man, his parents cut all ties with him. Merrill began taking hormone therapy and underwent gender confirmation surgery when he was 29.

Merrill decided to go to graduate school for social work. He found his calling working with troubled youth.

Merrill takes a multivitamin and a compounded herbal supplement every day. He has always been underweight. He has low blood pressure, so sometimes he gets dizzy when he stands up too quickly. Merrill's parents never talked much about their health when he was growing up. He would like to know if he has any genetic risk for chronic or serious diseases, but it is not worth trying to get in touch with them after all these years.

Merrill needs to find some type of exercise that will not cause too much discomfort in his neck and upper back.

Case Notes

Royce

Age: 22

Sex: Female

Race: Black

Occupation: Fitness Instructor

Royce is a bundle of energy. She teaches aerobics, power yoga, and dance at several health clubs. Once a week, she offers a free class on Instagram. Her teaching schedule has her on the go six days a week. She plans the routines and music for her classes and goes through her notes to remember the names of regular attendees. Royce recently hired a public relations consultant to help with her social media.

Royce works hard to take care of herself. She marks routines when she is teaching. That helps her focus on her students' body mechanics. It also minimizes risk that she will get too sore or injured.

Royce's workouts are usually very intense. She has never tried Pilates because she thinks it will not be challenging.

Royce's problem spots are her low back and calf muscles. These problems started when she was in a dance company in college. She worked with a physical therapist on corrective exercises and when to use heat or ice. If Royce is sore before teaching, she uses a topical analgesic. When she has had very tough days, she takes an over-the-counter pain reliever before going to bed.

Royce's mother is a former model. Her father works in real estate. Working out and staying fit was part of family life. Her older brother played club basketball and Royce took dance classes. Royce's maternal grandmother had trouble with vertigo all her life. Both of her grandfathers died in their sixties: one from colon cancer, the other from a heart attack. Her paternal grandmother has Type 2 diabetes.

Royce's commitment to fitness was inspired by her parents, and also by watching her beloved grandparents battle chronic diseases.

Case Notes

Oriana

Age: 47

Sex: Female

Race: Black

Occupation: Chef

Oriana has always loved to cook. One of her favorite possessions is a recipe binder she received for Christmas when she was 12. She used it to organize family recipes and recipes she cut out of the newspaper. Oriana was always experimenting in the kitchen.

Oriana studied political science in college. After she graduated, she worked for a consulting company. But Oriana missed cooking, so she diligently saved money with a plan to go to cooking school. Later, she met a chef who offered her a job in his kitchen. Oriana went to work for him and learned how to cook and run a restaurant. She eventually opened her own café.

After being on her feet all day, Oriana needs to stretch. She knows she also could benefit from core strengthening.

Oriana is prediabetic. She has had to change her diet and start eating less. That is difficult when she samples food in the kitchen. However, she tries to avoid desserts. When she gets tired at work, Oriana has a double espresso.

Oriana's father died of complications from kidney disease when he was 58. Her mother takes medication for hypertension and high cholesterol. Oriana's younger sister also has hypertension. With all of the chronic diseases in her family, Oriana is committed to taking care of herself.

When Oriana finds time to exercise, she usually feels good afterward. It also helps her get to sleep at night. A new Pilates studio opened up nearby. Oriana bought an introductory pack of three sessions to see what it is all about.

Case Notes

Kakie

Age: 39

Sex: Female

Race: Asian

Occupation: Realtor

Commercial real estate is the family business for Kakie. Both Kakie and her brother went to work for their father after graduating college and getting licensed. Kakie learned a lot about business from her father. She likes her job—especially because she can bring her dog to work.

So much of Kakie's life revolves around work. Meetings, site visits, dinners, and conference calls fill her days and sometimes her evenings. Networking is important to stay up-to-date on opportunities for her clients. Kakie finds time to work out with a personal trainer twice a week and belongs to a book club that meets once a month. Kakie and her brother have dinner with their parents every Sunday.

A few months ago, Kakie strained a groin muscle during a session with her trainer. She noticed tightness along her inner thigh right in the middle of a set on the adductor machine. The problem has gotten better, but the discomfort has not gone away.

Kakie has a vitamin D deficiency for which she takes a daily supplement. Her blood pressure and resting heart rate are normal, but she has never performed well on cardiovascular fitness tests. She has sensitive skin and is prone to breakouts but has no other health problems. Her grandparents are all still alive and healthy. Neither of her parents have chronic health problems, although her father smokes cigarettes. Kakie's brother takes medication for thyroid disease.

One of Kakie's clients rented space to a new Pilates studio. Kakie is considering adding Pilates to her weekly workouts with her trainer. She is not sure that Pilates will be challenging enough.

Case Notes

Jordan

Age: 31

Sex: Female

Race: White

Occupation: Retail Manager

Jordan is stressed. She just landed a job with a startup company that is launching luxury skincare products and fragrances. Jordan will be the district manager for a territory in the tristate area. This will be a step up the career ladder for Jordan. She is excited and nervous.

Jordan suffers from irritable bowel syndrome. She suffers from constipation and then has bouts of diarrhea that can last a day or two. Jordan's symptoms get worse when she is under a lot of stress. Often, the diarrhea episodes begin without any warning.

When Jordan first began experiencing symptoms, she saw her primary care provider, a gastroenterologist, a gynecologist, and a dietician. She changed her diet and kept a symptom log to try to identify food, activities, or anything that could contribute to the constipation or the diarrhea. She was advised to eat fiber and drink a lot of water; sometimes that made her feel bloated.

Jordan listens to music and tries to meditate for stress management. She tried to start running, but intense exercise exacerbates her symptoms. Jordan knows she needs to do some sort of exercise.

Jordan's mother has Type 1 diabetes. Meals were carefully planned when Jordan and her sister were growing up. Their mother always tried to be creative with proteins and vegetables. Jordan has not seen her father in years but is not aware that he has any health problems. Her sister suffers from migraines.

Jordan starts her new job next week. A gym near her new office offers Pilates. She is going to sign up for an introductory package of private sessions. Jordan wants to find some type of exercise that will help her get fit but not trigger her irritable bowel syndrome symptoms.

Case Notes

Noah

Age: 27

Sex: Male

Race: White

Occupation: Graduate Student

Noah is studying biology at a large university. Almost a year ago, he came down with mild flu-like symptoms a few weeks after returning from a research trip to northern Thailand. His skin was also itchy. He was diagnosed with acute hepatitis A infection. He followed recommendations from his primary care provider, but he was very tired. He had to rest a lot. It was difficult to keep up with his classes and work as a research assistant. His advisor was patient and let him complete some independent study work. Noah finally started to feel normal a month ago.

Noah broke his wrist when he was 13. He fell off a skateboard. He had his wisdom teeth removed when he was 17. He sees a dermatologist for acne rosacea. Other than that, Noah does not have any health problems. He tries to work out at the student recreation center a few times a week, but his schedule makes it difficult to find time. He generally grabs lunch at one of the restaurants on campus and gets takeout for dinner on his way home. When Noah was recovering from the acute hepatitis A infection, he ordered food for delivery because he was too tired to cook or go out. He gained a little weight.

Noah's father takes medication for hypertension and high cholesterol. Noah's mother is a breast cancer survivor. Noah has two sisters. The youngest was diagnosed a few years ago with late onset Tay-Sachs disease.

Noah feels like a lot of the past year was a fog. Now that he has some energy, he is thinking about starting some healthier habits. One of the other graduate students in his lab is a big fan of Pilates, so Noah is going to join her for a mat class.

Case Notes

Olga

Age: 43

Sex: Female

Race: White

Occupation: Certified Nursing Assistant

Olga hurt her back a few weeks ago lifting a patient. When it happened, she experienced a sharp pain in the middle of her back on the right side near her spine. She immediately went to the occupational health department at work where they had her rest and apply ice. She was scheduled for imaging tests the following day and advised to take an over-the-counter pain reliever.

When she woke the next morning, the middle of her back felt weak and achy. The imaging tests were inconclusive. She was diagnosed with nonspecific acute back pain.

Back pain is taken seriously in her department at work. Olga took leave of absence for a week. When she returned, she felt a dull ache and was on lifting restrictions.

Olga has been advised to try some gentle exercise to stretch and strengthen her back. Olga does not really like to exercise. The last time she had a gym membership, she felt lost in the weight room and had trouble following the routines in group aerobics classes.

Olga has trouble with her weight. She started to gain weight in her early twenties. She tried different diets to lose weight, but she always gained it back. Her blood pressure is normally high.

She is otherwise healthy. Both of her children were delivered by Caesarean section.

Olga is the youngest of six children. She has two brothers and three sisters. All of them have some type of chronic health problem: hypertension, diabetes, addiction. Her father died from kidney disease. Olga's mother has dementia and is in a long-term care facility.

The wellness program at work is going to start offering Pilates mat classes two nights a week. One of Olga's work colleagues convinced her to sign up.

Case Notes

Norman

Age: 42

Sex: Male

Race: White

Occupation: Pediatrician

Norman is a recreational rock climber. He climbs at a gym, takes day trips on weekends, and goes on climbing vacations with friends at least once a year. Norman loves climbing.

His left knee and ankle bother him occasionally. Years ago, when he was climbing at the gym, he fell off of a low hold. His climbing partner was not paying attention and did not react fast enough to pull up the slack in the rope. Norman landed hard on his feet and bit his tongue. He did not break any bones, but his legs and low back were sore for a few weeks. The left leg has bothered him ever since.

Norman always tries to stretch before and after climbing. He can usually muscle through when he gets sore, but sometimes ibuprofen or a topical analgesic are needed. When he takes a climbing trip, he always packs his first aid kit with some pain relievers. Other than this lingering discomfort, Norman does not have any health problems. He had his wisdom teeth removed under general anesthesia when he was 17. He has poor eyesight, so he always wears glasses or contact lenses.

Norman works at a pediatric urgent care clinic. His workdays can be hectic, but he finds his work interesting and rewarding rather than stressful. To unwind after a stressful day at the clinic,

Norman likes go to the climbing gym to workout and spend time with his friends.

Norman's father is also a physician and is a prostate cancer survivor. His mother has fibromyalgia. She has found that meditation and her support group help manage her symptoms.

Norman's leg discomfort does not affect his gait or ability to sleep. But he is annoyed that it is a lingering problem. A recent article about Pilates in a rock climbing magazine inspired Norman to sign up for a private session.

Case Notes

Layla

Age: 23

Sex: Female

Race: Pacific Islander

Occupation: Student

Layla is a part-time student at a community college. She is studying hospitality and tourism. She works weekends as a spa attendant at a resort. She has two younger brothers, so she also tries to help out her mother at home. Layla's dream is to open her own eco-tourism resort.

Layla has suffered from migraine headaches since she was in middle school. They seem to come on with no warning. It is very difficult for her to do anything when she has a migraine. She started taking prescription medication a few years ago which reduced the frequency of the migraines.

Other than migraines, Layla does not have any current health problems. She had a boating accident when she was in high school. Layla tripped when she and a friend were carrying a canoe. She fell forward, hit the canoe, and chipped her front teeth. Her teeth were repaired with veneers, and she has been fastidious about her oral health ever since.

Layla's father and mother are both a little overweight. Her mother also suffers from migraines. One of her younger brothers has autism spectrum disorder. Her paternal grandfather died from cancer, her maternal grandfather from heart disease. One of her grandmothers had angioplasty after she had a transient ischemic attack.

Layla met her boyfriend at the gym where he is a personal trainer. She usually works out towards the end of his shift so they can grab dinner together afterwards. The gym recently added a Pilates mat class. Layla usually does cardio and stacked weight machines. She is not sure that Pilates will be enough of a workout, but she is curious to try a class.

Case Notes

Rivkah

Age: 35

Sex: Female

Race: White

Occupation: Stay-at-Home Mother

Rivkah is a busy mother of five children. She stays organized with a family calendar. When her children are at school. Rivkah takes care of the housework and shopping. She loves to cook and enjoys trying new recipes. Her husband has a long daily commute to work at his family's business. Her days are full, but she tries to meet her older sister regularly for coffee or a manicure.

Rivkah has low back pain. It started when she was pregnant with her first child. When the pain bothers her, she takes an over-the-counter medication or uses a hot water bottle. Her primary care provider recommended that she exercise and lose weight, but Rivkah does not have time to exercise regularly. She does not like to exercise.

Rivkah's mother is a breast cancer survivor and her father has had atrial fibrillation for years. Her two sisters are both overweight. Rivkah's maternal grandmother died from pancreatic cancer. Her paternal grandmother died from breast cancer. Both of her grandfathers died from heart disease.

Rivkah's life is fulfilling. Even though she is busy, she rates her stress level as low. Her low back pain is sometimes an inconvenience, but it does not usually prevent her from doing anything. She notices that it bothers her with bending movements. She feels uncomfortable when she unloads the dishwasher, takes laundry out of the dryer, or ties her shoes.

One of Rivkah's friends started taking a Pilates class at the community center. She has been raving about how she feels taller and more aligned after class. She knows Rivkah has struggled with back pain and her weight and has been trying to convince Rivkah to join her for a class.

Case Notes

Mohammed

Age: 51

Sex: Male

Race: Asian

Occupation: Attorney

Mohammed loves playing soccer. He started playing almost as soon as he could walk. He played all through school and university. During high school, Mohammed sustained a concussion. He and another player hit each other when they were both trying to head the ball. Mohammed followed instructions to rest, but headaches and neck pain persisted for a long time. He also developed sensitivity to light. His friends teased him for wearing sunglasses most of the time.

His work as an intellectual property attorney involves a lot of sitting. He finds his work interesting but does not like sitting all the time. The only time Mohammed does not mind sitting is when he is watching his favorite teams on television. In the nice weather he stays active. Mohammed tries to kick a ball around the yard with his children after dinner. He plays in an adult recreational soccer league in the spring and summer. It is difficult to find things to do to be active when it is cold outside.

Mohammed was diagnosed with latent tuberculosis infection when he was in his early twenties. He recovered after following a medication regimen for almost a year. Other than that, the concussion, and an occasional knee sprain from playing soccer, Mohammed has not had any other health problems. His father died from lung cancer. His mother and sister do not have any current or chronic health problems.

Mohammed's wife has been trying to convince him to try Pilates. She takes a private session once a week and claims it has helped her back pain. Mohammed needs to find some activity to help him stay active during the cold weather.

Case Notes

Kalen

Age: 32

Sex: Male

Race: Black

Occupation: Musician

Kalen is a drummer and percussionist. He has collaborated with many well-known pop and jazz artists on recordings and performing. Kalen has toured all over the world. Kalen's life is music. He has been playing drums since he was seven years old.

Kalen's days are full of practicing and teaching lessons. On tour he teaches virtual lessons for his students. When he is rehearsing, recording, performing that involves a lot of late nights. He takes naps to ensure he gets adequate rest.

Kalen's work often involves business lunches or dinners. He tries to choose healthy items on the menu. Kalen runs to stay fit. When he packs to go on tour, his running shoes and a stretching strap are among the first few items that go into his suitcase. Running clears his head. Kalen enjoys exploring running routes in different cities. One of the artists Kalen toured with introduced him to golf. Kalen took some lessons and was hooked. He tries to play golf as often as he can.

When Kalen was at the music conservatory, he suffered from depression. Counseling and medication helped him recover. His therapist suggested that he try exercising. That is when Kalen started running. He joined a running group and made some new friends. It helped him feel better.

Part of Kalen's devotion to self-care comes from watching his parents battle chronic health problems. Kalen's father has Type 2 diabetes and his mother has hypertension. He has tried unsuccessfully to encourage them to exercise. But he did buy them fitness trackers and they try to get 10,000 steps every day.

The last artist Kalen toured with brought her Pilates equipment along on the road. She did Pilates every day. Kalen did not know anything about Pilates. After he got home he booked a session to see what Pilates was about.

Case Notes

Siobhan

Age: 27

Sex: Female

Race: White

Occupation: Copywriter

Siobhan is a copywriter for an advertising agency. She was recently promoted to a new account. This is an exciting opportunity for her, but it is also stressful. Stress aggravates her Crohn's disease symptoms.

Siobhan's gastrointestinal symptoms first emerged when she was in high school. She had bouts of abdominal pain and diarrhea and began to lose weight. After visits to various medical specialists and many diagnostic tests to rule out other conditions, Siobhan was diagnosed with Crohn's disease. Siobhan has had to figure out ways to manage her symptoms. She takes a combination of medications and has to carefully watch what she eats. Usually she eats small meals, but when her symptoms flare up, she fasts or eats a low-residue diet.

One of the things Siobhan has learned is that stress management is important. She made her apartment an oasis by decorating with soothing colors and scented candles. Regular walks in the park give her the opportunity to enjoy nature.

Siobhan's twin brother suffers from irritable bowel syndrome. Neither of their parents, nor any of their other siblings, has a gastrointestinal disorder. Their family has learned to be supportive of their dietary restrictions. But they do get teased for unusual food requests at family gatherings. Siobhan always asks for mashed potatoes and her twin brother requests banana pudding.

Siobhan's father has hypertension that is managed with medication. Her mother has neck problems related to osteoarthritis. One of her brothers has eczema. Her paternal grandfather died from liver cancer.

Siobhan made a resolution to start exercising. But she does not want to do anything too difficult. She is curious about Pilates and signed up for a trial session.

Case Notes

Catelyn

Age: 35

Sex: Female

Race: White

Occupation: Teacher

Catelyn is an elementary school teacher at a rural school. The close-knit community embraced Catelyn when she arrived five years ago. Although she missed the hustle and bustle of city life, Catelyn adapted to small town living in a way she never imagined.

Catelyn grew up in a suburb as the third of four children. Her family was very close and highly competitive. Like her sisters and brother, Catelyn excelled in sports. In high school she was president of the skiing club. She played on the lacrosse team in high school and college.

Catelyn injured her hip playing lacrosse. She strained her hip flexors and it never quite healed properly. Every so often. the pain flares up in her hip and low back. She takes an over-the-counter pain reliever and uses a heating pad in the evening. When her hip hurts, Catelyn has trouble sitting on the floor with her students during reading circles. She has even more difficulty getting up off the floor after a reading circle is finished. It has gotten worse over the years.

Catelyn's siblings had their fair share of sports injuries. Sprains and strains were so common, their mother always kept ice packs in the freezer and topical analgesics in the medicine cabinet.

None of them wanted to lose any practice or playing time. When Catelyn injured her hip, she had to sit out of lacrosse for two weeks. It was very difficult for her to watch from the sidelines. Out of all the injuries Catelyn sustained playing sports, the hip problem was the worst. She is annoyed that it still bothers her after all these years.

Catelyn is seeking new strategies to manage her hip problem. She wants to see if Pilates can help her move better and alleviate her discomfort in her hip.

Case Notes

Hannah

Age: 67

Sex: Female

Race: White

Occupation: Retired Sales Professional

Hannah retired a few years ago after a successful career as a sales representative for a beverage distributor. Since retiring, she has kept busy volunteering at a local food pantry and spending time with her grandchildren. Hannah and two of her friends have a subscription series to the opera and the orchestra. She also knits baby blankets for the local hospital

Hannah is a breast cancer survivor. She was diagnosed in her early fifties, and had a mastectomy and reconstructive surgery. The surgery left Hannah with limited range of motion in her shoulder. She feels fortunate that her cancer was caught early and that her treatment was successful. Her grandmother was not so lucky.

Hannah's mother also underwent treatment for a breast tumor that was found to be benign. Her mother is doing well in a long-term care facility and Hannah visits her weekly. Since breast cancer appears to have a genetic link, Hannah reminds her daughter to do monthly self-exams and get a routine mammogram.

Hannah's work in sales involved a lot of travel. Restaurant meals and lack of time to exercise contributed to weight gain. After Hannah finished treatment, she made a commitment to a healthy lifestyle. She used a smartphone app to log her meals and physical activity. Hannah made slow and steady progress to improve her fitness and lose weight. With time, she realized that she had more energy than she had in years.

One of Hannah's friends gave her some Pilates DVDs. She enjoyed the workouts and wants to learn more. She signed up for small group classes at a movement studio near her house.

Case Notes

Shanice

Age: 58

Sex: Female

Race: Black

Occupation: Physician Assistant

Shanice works in a small dermatology practice seeing a variety of patients. Most of her work involves treating common skin conditions and conducting skin cancer screenings, but the practice also offers cosmetic procedures. She works hard to develop a rapport with her patients. For Shanice, no two days are exactly alike.

Lately Shanice has been having tension-type headaches again. These are the same patterns of headaches she had after she gave birth to her first child. Back then, Shanice was a newlywed having difficulty with work-life balance. She left the large dermatology practice where she was working and took a position at a smaller practice. Over time, the headaches became less frequent.

No one else in her family has ever had the same trouble with headaches. The pattern of her headaches is always the same: a pain arches over her head from ear to ear and she feels tightness in her forehead and the back of her neck. Rest usually helps. If she gets a headache when she cannot rest, she takes an over-the-counter pain reliever and does neck and shoulder rolls to loosen the tension. Sometimes the headaches go away after an hour or two. Other times, they last until she goes to sleep at night.

For Shanice, the return of frequent headaches is inconvenient. When she has one at work, it is difficult to be present for her patients. When she has a headache at home, she is thankful that her husband will take care of things around the house until she feels better.

Shanice wanted to start a more regular exercise routine. She wants to start small group Pilates classes. She hasn't done Pilates in a long time but it always made her feel taller and more centered.

Case Notes

Leo

Age: 70

Sex: Male

Race: Black

Occupation: Retired Machinist

Leo retired seven years ago to care for his wife. She suffers from dementia and is unable to be left alone. She progressed from mild memory loss to severe symptoms over the course of two years. This decline was difficult for their whole family, but especially for Leo. They met when they were in high school. Watching her lose her memory is very sad.

His wife had been a stay-at-home mother. She took care of the children and all the housework. Leo had to learn how to become her caregiver and take care of their home. A local support group helped connect him with in-home services. She now has help twice a week with personal care. They receive respite care once a week so Leo can run errands and go shopping for groceries. Neither of their children live nearby, so Leo takes care of everything.

Leo's back has been bothering him. His support group stresses the importance of self-care. His back feels stiff and he does not want it to get worse.

Leo's work involved making parts out of metal and plastic. He was introduced to the machine shop through a vocational program in high school. He was intrigued by the fabrication process, worked hard, and was offered a job after he graduated.

He worked at the same machine shop for 44 years. His coworkers were like family.

Leo used to love going fishing. He looked forward to retiring so that he could spend more time on the water. Unfortunately, his wife's health declined, so instead of fishing, Leo is caring for her. He and his children feel it is important for her to stay in their home for as long as she can.

Leo wants to start exercising to help his back and his mental state. He will need to find a combination of something he can do on his respite days and then at home on his own. Someone in his support group takes Pilates at the gym and joins an online class when she needs to be at home. Leo thinks that might work for him too.

Case Notes

Skip

Age: 26

Sex: Male

Race: White

Occupation: Investment Banker

Skip's work as an investment banking analyst requires a lot of long days and many late nights. It is a competitive environment and Skip is determined to succeed. He knows that putting forth his best effort will help with his career development.

Skip is no stranger to competition. He is a former college football player. A key member of the defensive team, he still holds the school record for quarterback sacks. He started playing football in a peewee league and played every year from then until he graduated college. The most difficult part of college graduation was saying goodbye to football.

To be his best, Skip had to train hard. He credits his work in the weight room and a nightly stretching routine with keeping him healthy. Skip never sustained any major injuries in football.

Lately his back and knees have been bothering him. He takes an over-the-counter pain reliever and tries to stretch when he feels discomfort.

Skip works out at a gym three or four days per week. He feels comfortable in the weight room, so it helps him manage stress. He has put on a little weight. He blames meals ordered at work for the weight gain.

Skip's father was recently diagnosed with rheumatoid arthritis. He assumed the pain in his hands and wrists after playing tennis was from bad form. Medication is alleviating his symptoms. Skip's maternal grandparents died in a small plane crash when Skip was in high school. His paternal grandfather suffers from gout. Skip's mother, two sisters, and paternal grandmother are healthy. Skip jokes that the women in his family got a better set of genes.

One of Skip's favorite trainers at the gym is doing a Pilates teacher training course. He suggested that Skip try a few sessions.

Case Notes

Marque

Age: 27

Sex: Male

Race: Multiracial

Occupation: Model and Entrepreneur

Marque is a fit model for athletic and standard menswear. He tries on clothes for designers so they can check the draping, line, and appearance of new designs. When he has a fitting for athletic wear, he does simple exercises so the designer can see how the clothing moves. At each fitting, Marque models several different outfits, so he is changing clothes constantly.

Marque got his first job as a fit model when he was 19. His measurements were ideal for athletic wear. He branched out into standard menswear a few years ago.

Marque watches what he eats and works out every day to maintain his physique. He also pays close attention to how his clothes feel and checks his measurements on a regular basis. If he gains or loses weight, that interferes with how the designers can see their clothing.

On the side, Marque is developing his own skincare line. He has spent a long time searching for products that do not aggravate his sensitive skin. He hired a formulator and they are refining the sample products.

Marque is the baby of the family. He has two older sisters and an older half-brother. Their father was in the Army, so the family moved every few years when the children were growing up.

Moving was difficult but they all enjoyed living in different places.

Marque's father has hypertension; his mother has chronic obstructive pulmonary disease. His older brother has elevated blood pressure, so he is trying to change his eating and exercise habits. Marque has tried to support him.

Marque often has post-workout soreness. He was thinking about trying something new and saw a sign at the gym for an introduction to Pilates class.

Case Notes

Maya

Age: 51

Sex: Female

Race: White

Occupation: Nurse

Maya's back hurts all the time. It has been bothering her for years, especially after work. Maya works three twelve-hour shifts every week at the hospital. On her days off, she tries to rest, but she is often busy taking care of things around the house and making sure her children are keeping up with their schoolwork. Maya's extended family gets together most Sunday afternoons. However, she has missed a few gatherings because her back hurts.

Maya's back first started bothering her when she was pregnant with her first child. Over the years, pain flared up more frequently. Lately she has been in pain almost constantly. She has had a variety of imaging tests that did not find any structural reasons for her pain.

Maya needs relief from her back pain.

Maya and her husband are both overweight and have hypertension. They take daily medication and try to watch what they eat, but it is a challenge, especially at the Sunday family gatherings, because everyone brings food. Maya's parents also struggle with their weight and have hypertension. She suspects that these problems must be genetic.

Maya has three grandchildren that are the light of her life. She loves spending time with them, but it is difficult when her back hurts. Maya has been to physical therapy several times. It helped a little, but she does not remember the exercises anymore. She takes an over-the-counter pain reliever on a regular basis. She also uses a topical cream most nights before she goes to bed.

Maya's husband got her a gift certificate for a spa day at a nearby resort. When she called to schedule her spa services, the spa associate recommended starting her day with a Pilates mat class. Maya has never done Pilates before.

Case Notes

Ed

Age: 65

Sex: Male

Race: White

Occupation: Structural Engineer

Ed is quiet and methodical by nature. He approaches everything thoughtfully and logically, whether it is mowing the lawn, folding towels, or finding a parking space. Planning and attention to detail served him well in his work as a structural engineer. Ed is looking forward to retiring. He plans to plant a vegetable garden and go for long bike rides. Riding is one of his passions.

Ed is a prostate cancer survivor. He underwent successful treatment a few years ago. Just when he was getting back on his feet, his wife died suddenly after a ruptured brain aneurysm. Ed credits his children and the minister from his church with helping him through that very rough time.

Before his prostate cancer diagnosis, Ed was the picture of perfect health. He belonged to a local cycling club and rode with them most weekends. He and his wife were active in their church and played bridge once a month with other couples. Cancer treatment and his wife's death took a toll on Ed's physical and emotional health. His support network and riding were instrumental in helping Ed recover.

Ed's father died at age 58 from a heart attack and his mother died from emphysema when she was 72. Their health struggles inspired Ed to try to take better care of himself. Ed has one sister, but he does not speak to her because she is overweight and smokes cigarettes.

Both of Ed's children share his commitment to health. His son is also an avid cyclist and his daughter is a runner.

The tightness in his knees and hips has gotten a little worse lately. Ed notices it when he gets out of bed in the morning. One of his friends in the cycling club suggested that Ed try Pilates.

Case Notes

Eun-ji

Age: 54

Sex: Female

Race: Asian

Occupation: Bank Branch Manager

Eun-ji knows nearly everyone that comes into her suburban bank branch. She is on a first-name basis with the business account holders, home loan customers, and workers who come in to deposit their paychecks or purchase money orders.

Eun-ji has worked her way up to branch manager. When she started her career at the bank, Eun-ji had a wonderful boss. She learned a lot from him about developing relationships with customers. Her boss spent time chatting with regular customers. He also allowed dogs in the bank lobby and kept dog treats at the teller station. Eun-ji was afraid of dogs, but seeing customers with well-trained dogs in the bank helped her overcome her fear. Now Eun-ji even knows the names of her customers' dogs.

On weekends, Eun-ji takes care of household chores and spends time with her family. They enjoy playing tennis together. Her husband and two daughters are very competitive on the tennis court.

Eun-ji has been waking up lately with low back pain. She describes it as a stiffness and ache. She also notices the same discomfort at work when she stands up after sitting for a long time. Gentle stretching helps a little.

Eun-ji never remembers her parents ever being sick when she was growing up. They owned a small business and worked six days a week. To stay fit, they walked and got regular massages. When her father was diagnosed with lung cancer, her parents sold the business. He died a few months later. His illness took a toll on Eun-ji's mother. She started taking medication for hypertension and moved in with Eun-ji's sister.

Eun-ji wants to try to find something to loosen up stiffness in her back.

Case Notes

Yuri

Age: 39

Sex: Male

Race: White

Occupation: Architect

Yuri is a senior architect with a firm that specializes in theatres and performance spaces. His work is a combination of creativity and problem solving that relies heavily on teamwork. Yuri's even temper and calm demeanor is an asset in meetings with clients.

Yuri was diagnosed with Becker muscular dystrophy when he was 29. He first noticed weakness in his legs when he was playing golf. He mentioned it at an annual physical and his primary care provider ordered some tests. Very soon after that, Yuri was referred to specialists and underwent extensive medical testing. The diagnosis of Becker muscular dystrophy was a surprise to Yuri. He had never heard of this condition. He also did not know anything about his risk for genetic disease. Yuri was adopted as an infant and knows nothing about his birth parents.

After his diagnosis, Yuri tried to learn as much as he could about Becker muscular dystrophy. He discovered that it was important for him to exercise strategically. Yuri began working out to maintain strength in his legs and stave off deterioration of function. He does stationary cycling and uses weight machines four days a week. He is careful to keep his heart rate at a submaximal level when he cycles because of potential risks of damage to his heart muscles.

Yuri still plays golf every chance he gets. He follows a short stretching routine twice daily: after he wakes up in the morning and before bed at night. This alleviates discomfort and reduces muscle cramping.

Yuri also gets a brief massage every week as part of his wellness routine. One of his golf buddies just started taking Pilates group reformer classes and cannot stop talking about it. Yuri is curious to see what Pilates is all about.

Case Notes

Becky

Age: 42

Sex: Female

Race: White

Occupation: Pilot

Becky is a pilot for a private jet charter service. As a little girl, she always wanted to fly. She earned her pilot certificate at age 17 and has been flying ever since. Becky's job is as much about quality service as it is about flying. The company is a close-knit group. They pride themselves on customer service. The best part for Becky is that she gets to fly for a living.

Becky was diagnosed with breast cancer when she was just 31 years old. She found a lump during a monthly self-exam. It turned out to be malignant, so she underwent surgery, chemotherapy, and radiation treatment. She was very fatigued and lost all of her hair. She also had limited range of motion in her shoulder and edema in her arm. Becky was determined to regain her strength to get back into the air. She did extensive physical therapy for her arm after her cancer treatments ended.

Massage helped her regain range of motion in her shoulder and also helped her quality of life. She has gotten regular massages for her neck and shoulders ever since.

Breast cancer runs in Becky's family. Her mother and both of her grandmothers have been diagnosed with breast cancer. Because of her family history, Becky made sure to do her monthly self-exams. She feels lucky that she caught her cancer early.

Part of cancer survivorship for Becky involves working hard to stay healthy She meditates daily and runs 15 miles a week. Until recently she took tai chi class a few times a week. Becky's favorite tai chi instructor moved out of state. So Becky needs to find something new to replace tai chi. The movement studio where she took class also offers Pilates. Becky signed up for a group class.

Case Notes

Buck

Age: 30

Sex: Male

Race: White

Occupation: Data Scientist

Buck is a junior data scientist at a publishing company. He landed in this job after dropping out of graduate school and earning a certificate from a data bootcamp. Work is pretty confusing for Buck. He collects and cleans data, then passes it on to a data analyst. Communication about data in the company is not very clear. Often that means Buck has to do his work over again to include different variables. This is stressful for Buck.

Buck spends most of the day working at the computer. He tries to practice good posture, but his hands and wrists hurt. Buck got a cushion for his keyboard and a wrist rest on his mouse pad, but neither helped very much. He suspects it is carpal tunnel syndrome. The discomfort gets worse when Buck has to redo a work assignment. Stress aggravates Buck's wrists.

After Buck earned his undergraduate degree in biology, he was not sure what he wanted to do, so he got a job at a resort working as a ski instructor in the winter and hiking guide in the summer. After a few years, Buck decided to enroll in graduate school. He spent many hours in the lab working as a research assistant—and hated it. He saw an advertisement online for a data bootcamp. That seemed much more interesting than lab work. The pain in Buck's hands and wrists started after a few months at the publishing company.

In addition to focusing on his posture, Buck has been trying to stretch his shoulders, arms, and hands. He uses a topical analgesic a few times per day. Usually the pain is gone by the time he gets home after work.

Buck misses being fit. He wants to get back in shape so he can ski this winter. The movement studio across the street from the office posted a flyer for a package of introduction to Pilates sessions. Buck did an internet search about Pilates. What he found was very intriguing, especially the part about posture. Buck purchased a package and scheduled his first session.

Case Notes

Johanna

Age: 44

Sex: Female

Race: White

Occupation: Stay-at-Home Mother

Joanna is a former speech-language pathologist and current stay-at-home mother of two boys. She began to suffer from widespread muscle pain after the birth of her second child. She hoped to go back to work when her sons were in preschool, but pain and fatigue became persistent.

Joanna started taking over-the-counter pain relievers during the day and melatonin to get to sleep at night. However, she was still tired and in pain. She finally went to see her primary care provider. After a full physical, he referred her to specialists. Joanna underwent a series of tests and was diagnosed with fibromyalgia.

Joanna understands how chronic pain can affect a family. Her mother suffered from migraines for as long as Joanna can remember. Joanna and her sister had to help with cooking, cleaning, and laundry when their mother was unable to get out of bed. It was difficult for Joanna and her sister, but they grew close.

Her boys are too young right now to be of much help. Her husband works in the city and has a long commute. She struggles to take care of things at home and to stay awake to spend time with him after the boys are in bed. He has been very understanding, but Joanna is frustrated because she does not feel well most of the time.

Joanna has tried two prescription medications, but neither helped her pain. She still takes over-the-counter pain relievers and melatonin. She started listening to a meditation recording at night to help her get to sleep.

She read about a research study using exercise to help patients manage fibromyalgia. She is afraid to try anything intense like aerobics because she is worried that she will not be able to keep up. One of her friends goes to a small group class at a Pilates studio, she invited Joanna to join her to try Pilates.

Case Notes

Alice

Age: 24

Sex: Female

Race: Black

Occupation: Graduate Student

Alice is pursuing her MBA in marketing. She is currently in her second year of the program and just completed an internship with a large consumer packaged goods company. She hopes for an offer of a full-time position there after she graduates.

Most of her courses are interesting and all of them require a lot of reading. Alice tries hard to keep up. Many of Alice's courses involve group assignments. Thankfully, most of her classmates are responsible, so they get the work done. Still, the program is stressful, so Alice works out at the campus fitness center almost daily to help manage stress.

Lately, her low back has been bothering her, especially when she has been sitting for a long time. Standing up after a lecture can be painful. Her back also feels stiff when she gets out of bed in the morning. Alice's back does not usually bother her when she is working out. That may be because she always makes sure to warm up before exercise. Alice has been able to link the back pain with sitting and being still for a very long time.

Alice's father was recently diagnosed with kidney cancer. Luckily, his cancer was found early. But back pain was one of his symptoms, so Alice is anxious about her own back pain. Alice's mother told her to keep a diary of her back-pain symptoms to monitor if the pain patterns were consistent or worsened and make an appointment with the student health center to make sure the pain is not linked to a larger problem.

Alice followed her mother's advice, but she also signed up for a Pilates mat class at the fitness center. She read an article that it can help back pain. She is willing to try anything.

Case Notes

Joe

Age: 68

Sex: Male

Race: White

Occupation: Mechanic

Joe and his wife own a busy automotive repair shop. She handles the office and he works on cars. They have worked together for over forty years and raised three children. Their son now works in the shop and will inherit the family business if Joe ever decides to retire.

Joe almost retired seven years ago. He was diagnosed with Stage 1 lung cancer. That was a scary time. Joe had chemotherapy and radiation treatments and the tumors disappeared. He still has regular scans to make sure the cancer has not come back.

Joe has never smoked, so the lung cancer diagnosis was a big surprise. His oncologist thought that all of the years Joe spent working around gas and oil in repair shops might have exposed him to some chemicals that increased his cancer risk. As a cancer survivor, Joe made a commitment to take care of his health.

When Joe was undergoing treatment at the cancer center, he met with a dietician to review his meal habits and make healthy changes. Now Joe and his wife bring lunch from home to work every day. Joe calls the soups and salads "rabbit food," but he knows they are healthier for him than deli sandwiches from the place up the street. Joe and his wife try to walk 10,000 steps every day and wear fitness tracker to measure their progress.

With the fitness tracker "gadget" and the "rabbit food" Joe has been successful with lifestyle changes.

Joe's wife has been taking a small group Pilates class weekly for a long time. She is usually in a good mood and standing up a little taller after class. Recently Joe's neck started bothering him. It is stiff after a long day at the shop. He has tried warm compresses and stretching but that only helps a little. His wife has convinced him to sign up for an introductory small group class at the Pilates studio.

Case Notes

Armando

Age: 40

Sex: Male

Race: White

Occupation: Police Officer

Armando joined the village police force after serving in the Navy. His wife grew up nearby, they moved to the village to raise their children after he left the Navy. Working in a small department in a small town means that Armando knows everyone. On or off shift, he regularly visits local stores and restaurants to maintain good relationships with business owners. Armando also gives safety presentations at the local elementary school every year. He enjoys small town life.

Armando struggles with his weight. He has been on blood pressure medication for a few years and was recently told he is prediabetic. Armando's back also hurts a lot of the time.

Armando's son started playing in a baseball league and aspires to be an outfielder. Armando wants to help him practice fielding baseballs. A week ago, when they were at the park, Armando felt a sharp pain in his back. The pain has lessened, but has not gone away entirely.

Armando needs to get rid of his back pain so he can play ball with his son.

Armando's mother and grandmother both have diabetes. His father died from heart disease. Armando recognizes that he needs to take better care of his health. He recently joined a health education program at the community center. His group is working with a diabetes educator on lifestyle modifications. They have had sessions on cooking, exercise, and stress management. Armando has not really learned anything new in the program, but it does provide a reminder that he can take care of his health by changing his habits.

The community center is offering an introduction to Pilates workshop. Armando wonders if that would help his back pain.

Case Notes

Gabriella

Age: 56

Sex: Female

Race: White

Occupation: Small Business Owner

Gabriella owns a successful janitorial business. She launched her commercial cleaning business fifteen years ago with a minority and women-owned business grant. Her staff cleans offices in several of the largest buildings in town. She has worked hard to grow the business and support her staff. Many of her employees have worked at the company for years.

Gabriella is a Rotarian, active in her church, and volunteers once a month at a local women's shelter. Close ties to her community help her feel fulfilled and also have helped her succeed as a businesswoman. Gabriella has a lot of meetings with regular clients, potential clients, vendors, and administrative staff. She also conducts regular site visits to ensure her employees' work exceeds standards.

About a year ago Gabriella's husband had a health scare. It encouraged him to make some lifestyle changes. He now exercises regularly, tries to walk 10,000 steps a day, and is working on stress management. His positive changes have inspired Gabriella to prioritize her own health.

When Gabriella in her early twenties, she was in a car crash. She was a passenger in a taxi that was hit by another car. She sustained a fractured cheekbone and contusions on her face. She healed completely, except for a small scar on the side of her face. It is barely noticeable anymore. She has no health problems, other than bunions from years of wearing high-heeled shoes, Gabriella is a little overweight. She does not exercise but is always on the go.

A movement studio near Gabriella's office posted a sign that it is under new management. They are offering discounted introductory packages for new clients. Gabriella has always been curious about Pilates.

Case Notes

Santiago

Age: 41

Sex: Male

Race: White

Occupation: Engineer

Santiago is a mechanical engineer. He currently works on a private yacht. His work takes him all over the world, so Santiago has seen some beautiful places. His job is to keep the yacht running smoothly. Santiago loves to travel, and he is fascinated by all things mechanical. He is lucky to have found the perfect job to suit his interests and talents.

Santiago earned a soccer scholarship to college. He majored in mechanical engineering with the hope of getting a job in manufacturing. But instead, he met a cousin of one of his soccer teammates who worked as a deckhand in the yachting industry. Santiago always wanted to see the world. After graduating from college, he got a job on a yacht and worked his way up.

Some of Santiago's work requires contorting himself into small spaces. Every so often, he feels a twinge in his back. He stretches and ices to help it feel better and sometimes gets a massage to alleviate discomfort.

Playing soccer helped Santiago develop some healthy habits. He still tries to stay fit. Santiago watches what he eats, does calisthenics every day, and tries to go for a run when the yacht is in port. Living in small quarters with the other crew members can be difficult at times. For Santiago, exercise helps him with stress management.

Both of Santiago's parents and his older sister take medication for hypertension. His father is pre-diabetic. Several of his other relatives have diabetes. Santiago knows that the family history probably increases his risk for hypertension and diabetes. He is committed to trying to take care of his health to reduce risk of chronic diseases.

Santiago feels like he needs to take his back problem a bit more seriously. One of his crewmates suggested he add Pilates mat exercises to his routine.

Case Notes

Quinn

Age: 29

Sex: Male

Race: American Indian

Occupation: Firefighter

Quinn is a career firefighter in a large metropolitan department. He finished his probationary period and was assigned to an engine company downtown. Quinn enjoys the camaraderie of the firehouse. He finds the work challenging and rewarding.

Lately, Quinn's right knee has been bothering him. He notices pain when he walks downstairs and when he steps down off the engine after a call. He rarely notices it any other time when he is at work.

Quinn works out in the fire station gym on every shift, lifting weights and riding the stationary bicycle. He is not very good at remembering to stretch. On his days off he goes running with his dog. When the weather is nice they explore trails in a large park. For Quinn the combination of nature, running, and being with his dog are the perfect way to spend a morning. The only time his knee bothers him is when he runs down hills.

Quinn was a running back on his high school football team. The coaching staff worked with the students on weight training programs. Quinn still follows the same full-body workout sequence he learned back then. He likes the familiarity of the routine.

Quinn's mother has asthma and suffers from diabetes. She has struggled with her weight for as long as Quinn can remember. His father died in an accident when Quinn was 15. Quinn's maternal grandmother had very bad osteoarthritis in her knee and hip. Quinn wonders if osteoarthritis is hereditary.

Quinn gets an annual physical with the fire department. Other than the occasional knee pain, he is in good health.

The fire department fitness center recently started offering a group Pilates class. The focus is on helping firefighters with back pain but it is open to anyone in the department.

Case Notes

Melissa

Age: 48

Sex: Female

Race: Black

Occupation: Nurse

Melissa is a perioperative nurse at a regional hospital. She was an Army nurse and served several tours overseas. When she left the military, Melissa moved back to her hometown to be near her mother. She easily landed a job at the hospital. Her job as a perioperative nurse leverages her skill set. She works for an orthopedic surgeon to prepare patients for surgery, monitor them during surgery, and follow up with them afterwards. Melissa's colleagues admire her confident and professional demeanor.

Melissa's low back has been bothering her again. She has had pain on and off over the years. It is always the same type of deep muscle ache. At various times she has taken medication, gone to physical therapy, and tried different exercise programs. The ache goes away, but eventually it comes back.

Melissa was an athlete growing up. She played on her high school basketball team and played intramural volleyball in college. She jogs 10-12 miles a week, mostly to clear her head. Melissa always stretches after she runs.

Melissa's mother was diagnosed with colon cancer at age 72. She had surgery and chemotherapy. She is now in remission; her recent scans were clear. Her father died of a heart attack when he was just 53 years old. Melissa's brother is overweight and has hypertension. She nags him often to take better care of his health.

Over the years, Melissa has developed her own protocol to deal with her back pain. She does a series of stretches twice a day and applies a heat pack at night. When it hurts at work, Melissa takes ibuprofen and uses a topical analgesic.

She has been getting bored with her stretching routine. Melissa read an article about Pilates and back pain. It sounds interesting and worth trying.

Case Notes

Benjamin

Age: 41

Sex: Male

Race: White

Occupation: Robotics Technician

Benjamin loves robotics. When he was growing up, he was in the robotics club at school. He and his friends designed and built robots that could perform a variety of functions. Benjamin's favorite design was a remote-control robot that could carry a cup of coffee across the classroom to his teacher.

Benjamin achieved his goal to study engineering in college. After graduating, he started working at a biomedical engineering company. He works on modular limbs that are used as prosthetics for individuals who have had an amputation. Benjamin's job is interesting—and it can make a difference in the lives of amputees.

Benjamin is a testicular cancer survivor. When he was 23, he suddenly felt dizzy and fell when he was at the mall. The mall security department insisted that he go to the emergency room where it was discovered that he had a brain tumor. Testicular cancer had metastasized. Benjamin underwent successful treatment and has been cancer free ever since.

Benjamin has been vigilant about his health ever since that day at the mall. He feels vulnerable. He keeps a headache diary to monitor his symptoms because he learned that a change in headache patterns might signal a problem. He also follows his oncologist's advice to manage stress.

Benjamin and his wife have a stationary bicycle and a rowing machine in their basement. They both try to do a cardio workout every other day. Benjamin has been getting bored with the routine. He read an article about Pilates and found the pictures of the equipment fascinating. He is curious to know more about the designs and how the springs work. Much to his wife's surprise, Benjamin scheduled an introductory session at a Pilates studio near their house.

Case Notes

Liliana

Age: 39

Sex: Female

Race: White

Occupation: Hair Stylist

Liliana owns a local franchise of a specialty salon designed to help children have fun getting haircuts. Her salon looks like a cross between a play space and a workplace. Everything is brightly-colored. The stations have toys for the children to sit on instead of styling chairs. The waiting area has a small playground. Liliana loves the cheerful environment.

Liliana's friendly nature has helped her grow her business. She has given families tours of the salon, let children practice sitting in the styling "chairs," and explained the process of a haircut. Liliana is dedicated to customer service for the whole family. She has earned a reputation for being successful with even the most difficult little clients.

Sometimes Liliana gets a stiff neck when she works. It is more of a tightness than pain but it is uncomfortable. A massage usually helps. But Liliana thinks she might need to improve her posture.

When Liliana was growing up, her mother had very bad osteoarthritis in her spine. It bothered her a lot. Her mother had a traction device that she was supposed to use every day. If she did not use the traction, the pain would flare up. Liliana's mother did not like to take pain medication, so she would ask Liliana to massage her neck. Over the years, the pain never seemed to get better or worse. Her mother had to learn how to manage the pain.

Because of her mother's medical history, Liliana thought she might also have osteoarthritis, but so far, she does not. That means her stiff neck is probably tension or poor posture. Liliana knows she should exercise and eat better. But it is difficult because the salon is so busy. Stretching would probably help when her neck gets stiff.

One of Liliana's stylists started taking a Pilates group class. She has been raving about how good she feels after a workout. Liliana is curious to know if Pilates could help her posture and neck problem.

Case Notes

Annette

Age: 75

Sex: Female

Race: White

Occupation: Retired Professor

Annette is a scholar of deviant behavior. She is best-known for her work on marital infidelity. She taught at a large university and lectured all over the world. Although she retired from the university, Annette still writes articles and gives interviews. Her work is her hobby.

Years ago, Annette was diagnosed with osteoporosis. She developed problems with hips and knees. Eventually she had joint replacement surgery for both of her hips and her right knee. Navigating the campus was tricky while she recovered from each surgery, but she tried to exceed the rehabilitation recommendations and that helped her recovery.

Even though she is retired, Annette still spends most of her day at her desk in her home office. She finds that she needs to stretch after she has been sitting for a long time. Lately her back has been bothering her.

Annette takes medication and a dietary supplement for her osteoporosis. She also takes a multivitamin every day. Since retiring, Annette goes for a long walk every morning. She also attends tai chi class a few times a week at the local senior center. Annette was never much of an exerciser, but she has noticed that practicing tai chi has improved her balance.

Annette's husband died three years ago after suffering a stroke. They were married for 37 years. Annette and her husband had a standing invitation to spend holidays with her niece. Annette has continued that tradition. But her niece also calls her every Sunday, just to check in. Between her regular chats with her niece, interactions at the senior center, and an occasional interview, Annette feels that she has a good amount of social interaction.

Annette has never tried Pilates. She read an article about Pilates and back pain and thinks it is worth trying.

Case Notes

Ziggy

Age: 27

Sex: Transgender

Race: White

Occupation: Bartender

Ziggy tends bar at a beach resort. They serve a lot of beer and wine coolers but also gets to make fun, fancy cocktails most days. Ziggy has fun making intricate arrangements of fruit and edible flowers on skewers to garnish drinks.

The resort grounds are lush and tropical. The beautiful environment helps make up for the occasional rude guest or poor tipper. The owners of the resort invest heavily in training for all employees. New employee orientation is extensive. Everyone is required to attend training sessions before the start of the regular tourist season. When Ziggy started working at the resort, required attendance at training sessions seemed onerous. But Ziggy has learned a lot about hospitality and service. Strategies for communication and problem solving have been especially helpful in dealing with resort guests.

Low back pain has become a problem for Ziggy. The dull ache and stiffness at the end of a shift is almost guaranteed. Ziggy was referred to occupational health for evaluation. Imaging tests did not reveal any structural problems.

Ziggy's mother always had back pain. She worked for a commercial laundry service. For years, her job involved pulling and pushing large bins around the plant or operating the automatic folding machine. Eventually she was promoted to an account manager. Her back pain got better but it never really went away. She learned to manage it.

Ziggy's mother suggested trying a topical analgesic before work and icing or using a heat pack after work. Her recommendations helped a little, but Ziggy needs to find better solutions.

One of the waitstaff found Pilates to be helpful to deal with a shoulder problem. She suggested Ziggy try Pilates.

Case Notes

Jeff

Age: 40

Sex: Male

Race: White

Occupation: Art Director

Jeff works in the creative department for a retail clothing chain. He collaborates with designers and copywriters on branding, layout, and seasonal installations. These days, Jeff spends most of his time at work in meetings. When he was an assistant art director, he spent nearly all of his time at a drafting board or computer. His job back then was executing someone's vision. Now, he works as part of the team that develops the vision. But some days, Jeff misses the solitude of drawing and retouching photographs.

When he was growing up, Jeff wanted to be a professional photographer. But when Jeff was in art school, he got an internship at a clothing company. He realized that type of job would provide more stability. Jeff still takes photographs for a hobby. When he and his girlfriend go to the park, zoo, or botanical garden on weekends, Jeff always brings his camera. He shares his photos on social media and has built a nice following.

Five years ago, Jeff had acute abdominal pain and ended up in the hospital. The doctors suspected that his pain was appendicitis, but it turned out to be an umbilical hernia. They were surprised because he did not have the typical risk factors. He had an emergency surgery and it took a long time for him to recover. Because Jeff rarely gets sick, surgery and being hospitalized was a very stressful experience. He was able to recover at home and work remotely while he regained strength.

After the experience with the hernia, Jeff resolved to start a self-care program. He writes a daily journal, tries to eat a healthy diet, and gets a monthly massage. He knows he needs to start exercising, but finds the weight room at the gym uninspiring. His girlfriend really enjoys Pilates and offered to treat Jeff to a session with her Pilates teacher.

Case Notes

Margaret

Age: 59

Sex: Female

Race: White

Occupation: Music Teacher

Margaret is a piano teacher. She is part-time faculty at a community college and also teaches piano lessons in her home. Margaret started playing piano when she was six years old. Growing up, Margaret gave recitals and accompanied the school choirs. She majored in music education in college and taught high school music until she got married. After her third child was born, Margaret was offered a part-time teaching job at the community college. Ever since, Margaret has taught 15-20 private lessons a week during the school year.

Margaret has struggled with her weight ever since she had children. She tries to watch what she eats, but does not like to exercise. Walking a lot bothers her left hip and low back.

Margaret had back pain during each of her three pregnancies. She tried prenatal yoga and it helped a little. The back pain never really went away. Some days it is worse than others. Margaret briefly kept a pain diary to try to identify what sorts of things might trigger the pain but she was never able to figure anything out.

Margaret knows she is lucky that she is able to sit when she teaches lessons. However, walking from her car to the music building at the community college can be painful.

Most nights, Margaret uses a heat pack or hot water bottle on her back. She has a prescription for a pain reliever, but she tries not to take it because it makes her groggy.

Margaret knows that exercise could help her lose weight and might help her back and hip problems. She is self-conscious about being overweight and is reluctant to go to a group exercise class. A story in the newspaper about a Pilates studio that opened a new location looked interesting because they offer private sessions.

Case Notes

Hwan

Age: 57

Sex: Female

Race: Asian

Occupation: Hotel Concierge

Hwan works for a large hotel chain at the concierge desk. She makes reservations at restaurants, tourist attractions, and helps guests find fun and interesting things to do in her city. Hwan tries to keep up with news and events so she can be well-informed for hotel guests.

Hwan's parents owned and operated a bed and breakfast, so Hwan grew up in the hospitality business. While she was working on an associate's degree in hospitality and tourism, Hwan did an internship at a large hotel chain. She was offered a concierge job immediately after finishing her degree. Hwan's parents sold the bed and breakfast a few years ago. They hoped that Hwan would take over the business, but Hwan has enjoyed her life in the city too much to ever move back home.

Hwan had a seizure when she was 14 years old. It happened without any warning. She had not been ill or sustained any injuries. She just had a seizure one day at school. Not long after that, she had another seizure. Hwan had a series of medical tests and was ultimately diagnosed with epilepsy. She started taking medication and following a ketogenic diet.

Although Hwan cannot be sure, being stressed might be a trigger for seizures. She makes stress management a priority. She does breathing exercises and journaling every morning, and gets occasional massages. Hwan like to sample the various spas and fitness centers near the hotel so she can make recommendations to guests.

Recently several guests have wanted to book Pilates sessions. Hwan found a few options for private appointments and group classes at studios near the hotel. She wants to try a few sessions to get insights that can help her work as a concierge.

Case Notes

Valeria

Age: 25

Sex: Female

Race: White

Occupation: Teacher

Valeria teaches fifth-graders at an elementary school in an underserved area. She grew up in the neighborhood and wanted to give back to her community after she earned a scholarship to college. Valeria was thrilled to land a job at the same school she attended. Although the neighborhood has changed a little, Valeria still feels very much at home.

Valeria lives with her mother and grandmother. At first it was strange to move back home after college, but they can all save money and Valeria does not have to commute to school. Plus, her grandmother cooks and cleans the apartment so Valeria is somewhat spoiled.

Other than walking half a mile to school and back every day, Valeria makes little effort to exercise. She spends most of her evenings grading student assignments and refining lesson plans for the following day. If her grandmother did not cook, Valeria probably would not take time for dinner.

Valeria is prediabetic. Her mother and grandmother both have diabetes. Not long ago, Valeria talked with a health educator at a community health fair. She learned that changing her diet could help her diabetes. For Valeria, that would be difficult because she would need to refuse her grandmother's meals. The health educator gave Valeria a flyer for a healthy cooking class. Valeria is trying to drum up courage to give the flyer to her grandmother. She wants to find a way to talk with her mother and grandmother about diabetes. She is concerned about the long-term effects it will have on their health.

The health educator recommended that Valeria start a regular exercise program. She joined a gym in the neighborhood and had a few orientation sessions with a personal trainer. The group exercise classes look like they might be more fun than the weight machines and cardio equipment. Valeria is trying to convince herself to try the Pilates class.

Case Notes

Jiro

Age: 41

Sex: Male

Race: Asian

Occupation: Investment Banker

Jiro is a managing director at a small investment bank. His firm specializes in the food and beverage industry. When Jiro started out as an analyst, he worked very long days at a large firm. He pursued his MBA through an executive program. His hard work paid off as he received promotions. Jiro now manages a team of associates and analysts. When they are working on a deal, he still has to put in long hours, but he also gets to meet with clients and travel more than junior members of his team.

Jiro goes to the gym every morning before work. When he travels he always works out in the hotel gym. He does cardio workouts or weight training on alternate days. He and his wife play in a mixed doubles tennis league in the summer. Jiro likes to stay fit and he enjoys competition.

Sometimes Jiro has low back pain. When his back hurts gentle movement and stretching usually helps him feel a little better. But Jiro has always had tight hamstring muscles. When he was in elementary school, he always did poorly on the stretching component of fitness tests. Jiro was a good student, but he never could figure out how to ace the fitness test.

Jiro's father is a retired investment banker and avid golfer. He also suffers from back pain and had a lumbar discectomy when he was in his fifties. He learned a short exercise and stretching in rehabilitation and does it every day. He often nags Jiro about the importance of stretching.

Jiro has a membership to a massage clinic. He gets a massage once a month. He likes the massage therapist to focus on his back. He usually feels good for a few days afterwards. His wife started taking private Pilates sessions and thinks it would be good for Jiro.

Case Notes

Alejandro

Age: 38

Sex: Male

Race: White

Occupation: Commercial Fisherman

Alejandro works as a foreman on a commercial fishing boat. He started out in the industry as a deckhand on his uncle's boat. Alejandro worked his way up on the crew by learning different types of jobs. During the season the days are very long and the crew lives in tight quarters. The work is messy, but the money is good, and Alejandro loves being on the water. He lives on the boat to work a season and then gets to go home in the off season to spend time with his wife and children.

Alejandro has a chronic injury to his right shoulder. The problem started when he tore a rotator cuff muscle lifting a net. An MRI revealed a tear. His doctor recommended physical therapy instead of surgery. The combination of exercises, stretches, and massage helped Alejandro strengthen his shoulder muscles and retain full range of motion. For the most part it was successful, but occasionally Alejandro feels a twinge of pain when he moves a certain way. That pain reminds him to be careful.

Other than the shoulder problem, Alejandro is relatively healthy. He lifts weights during the off season so he can stay fit for his work on the boat. He has to be careful doing overhead lifts so he does not hurt his shoulder. He is a little overweight. He likes to eat and drinks beer occasionally. Alejandro's maternal grandfather died from lung cancer, so Alejandro has never smoked.

Alejandro knows that he needs to stay healthy so he can work and provide for his family. He is thinking that changing up his workout routine might be helpful. His gym started offering group Pilates reformer classes. Alejandro heard Pilates was helpful for core strength and back pain, but he is not sure it will be good for his shoulder.

Case Notes

Shirley

Age: 52

Sex: Female

Race: White

Occupation: Veterinarian

Shirley owns a suburban veterinary practice. She primarily sees cats and dogs, but her clients also have rabbits, guinea pigs, and hamsters. Most of Shirley's workdays involve routine examinations and vaccinations, except Tuesdays. She does scheduled surgeries on Tuesdays. A year ago, an emergency veterinary facility opened up a few miles away. Originally, Shirley was worried about her business, but the emergency facility is only open evenings and weekends, so that ended up being helpful for Shirley. She sends her patients to them and they refer back to her.

Shirley has eczema. She gets patches on her forearms year-round, and her legs in the winter. Her dermatologist suspects that it started with an allergic reaction to something. Shirley washes her hands a lot at work. Her office recently switched to hypoallergenic soap and cleaning products and hopes that might help. Shirley also uses prescription cream on affected areas, and that helps a little. Shirley gets regular massages to alleviate tension in her neck and upper back.

Shirley was always athletic. She went to an all-girls high school where she played on the volleyball and basketball teams. In college she played intramural sports. Both of her daughters play soccer. Shirley's Saturday mornings are usually spent on the sidelines of a field cheering them on. Her youngest daughter has patches of eczema on her legs. She also suffers from asthma. Shirley's mother also had asthma, so they suspect it runs in the family.

The tension in her neck and upper back has been a little worse lately. Shirley thinks that it might be time to change up her exercise routine. She has only done Pilates mat classes and has never tried in apparatus session. She wonders in it would be good or bad for her neck.

Case Notes

Lorenzo

Age: 58

Sex: Male

Race: White

Occupation: Dentist

Lorenzo is a family dentist. His father was also a dentist. Lorenzo joined him in the family practice. After his father retired, Lorenzo took over the practice. They are well-known in their community and have treated several generations of the same families.

Lorenzo suffers from nonspecific back pain. He has never sustained any injuries to his back. While he has always been active, he was never an athlete. He has visited specialists and had a variety of imaging tests. The results have all been inconclusive. He was prescribed pain medication, but never filled the prescription. Lorenzo was worried about addiction. One of his friends became addicted to opioids when they were prescribed after surgery.

For his back pain, Lorenzo takes an over-the-counter pain reliever and uses a heat pack at night. Lately, his back pain has been more persistent, and he has had trouble sleeping. It is not because of the pain itself but because he is worried about the pain. Worry keeps him awake.

Lorenzo's orthopedist mentioned that stress and back pain can be related, so he recommended that Lorenzo focus on stress management. For Lorenzo, the best therapy is working on his coin collection. He has been an avid coin collector since he was a child. He finds it very therapeutic to do the detailed work required to organize his collection. He enjoys attending numismatic lectures. At least once a year, he travels to a show.

Lorenzo's father also suffered from back pain but his was due to degenerative disc disease. Lorenzo is hoping to avoid the same fate.

Lorenzo also occasionally gets a massage for pain relief. He keeps hearing about Pilates and is curious to give it a try. He wants to know if it could help his back pain.

Case Notes

Fabiana

Age: 29

Sex: Female

Race: Black

Occupation: Designer

Fabiana fell in love with home fashion when she was 10 years old and her family moved from a small apartment into a house. Her mother thoughtfully decorated one room at a time. She had a strict budget, so she and Fabiana went to discount stores, resale shops, and garage sales to find furnishings for their house. Fabiana loved collaborating with her mother to turn their house into a home. It inspired Fabiana to want to study design.

Fabiana won a scholarship to college to study art and design. After graduation, she got a job as a fabric designer. She studies current and upcoming trends in colors and patterns to design fabrics. She specializes in fabric for home furnishings. She works long hours drawing by hand and then plotting out patterns using a computer program. Most of her days are spent sitting at her desk. By lunchtime, she usually has a stiff neck. By the end of the day, she often has a headache. Despite feeling uncomfortable after work Fabiana loves her job.

Both of Fabiana's parents have musculoskeletal problems. Her father has always had back pain. He is an executive director for a nonprofit organization and always seems to be stressed. He has had many x-rays and even MRIs that did not find anything wrong with his back. Fabiana often wondered if his work stress was linked to his back pain. Fabiana's mother has lupus. She has widespread pain and has been trying to get it under control for years. Massage sometimes helps.

One of Fabiana's friends just got certified in Pilates and is opening a business. She wants Fabiana to come take a class. Fabiana is not sure whether it will make her neck feel better or worse but she wants to support her friend.

Case Notes

Chiyoko

Age: 37

Sex: Female

Race: Asian

Occupation: Software Engineer

Chiyoko is a former elite athlete. As a long-distance runner, she competed in marathons and half marathons until she was sidelined with a hip injury. When she had to stop running, Chiyoko went back to college to pursue a second bachelor's degree in computer science. After finishing, she landed a job at a tech startup. She has worked at a series of startups. The hours can be long, but financially, it is very rewarding.

Chiyoko is a single mother. Her six-year-old daughter is her pride and joy. Chiyoko shows everyone she meets pictures on her phone of her daughter doing something cute. According to the divorce agreement, Chiyoko and her ex-husband were supposed to split custody of their daughter, but he remarried, and he and his new wife have twins. Chiyoko is angry at his claims he is too busy to see his daughter, but she is secretly happy. Whenever he cancels his custody visits it gives her more time with her daughter.

Chioyoko's hip still bothers her after all these years. When she was running competitively, she stretched and got massages. Even though she isn't running she needs a strategy to help with pain and range of motion.

Chiyoko's father was also an elite athlete. He started her running when she was in elementary school. She was proud to watch him compete in races and loved when he came to cheer her on at track meets. He was fortunate to never suffer any major injuries during his running career. After retiring, he became a financial planner.

One of Chiyoko's friends offered her a buddy pass for a new class at a Pilates studio. Chiyoko is curious. She wonders if she would be able to do the exercises given the lingering problems with her hip.

Case Notes

May

Age: 59

Sex: Female

Race: Black

Occupation: Bookkeeper

May has run a successful bookkeeping business for over 30 years. She started her business because she needed a flexible work schedule when her children were young. May grew the business based upon referrals from clients. It blossomed into more than she could have imagined when she started out.

May works out of her home office. First thing in the morning, she organizes her calendar. Her last task at the end of her workday is tidying up her desk and files. May works best when her office is in order. Although she meets with clients by phone or video conference, most of her day is spent with numbers, spreadsheets, receipts, and file folders. May finds structure comforting.

May's feet and legs often cramp at night. Lately it has gotten a little worse. Getting out of bed and stretching is the only thing that provides relief. May and her husband are both prediabetic. Her A1C level has hovered around 6% for a while. They both know that diet and exercise modification can reduce their diabetes risk, but change is difficult. Her husband works long hours so May takes care of the food shopping and meal preparation. She loves to cook family favorites, especially when her sons come home to visit.

Last year for Christmas, one of their sons got May and her husband wearable activity trackers. The novelty of competing with each other for the most steps every day quickly wore off, but they did start a new habit of taking walks around the neighborhood after dinner. It has not helped May lose any weight, but she enjoys the relaxing time with her husband.

May is thinking that she needs to find a new strategy for exercise that will not make her leg cramps worse. She read an article in a magazine about Pilates and wants to try class.

Case Notes

Alanna

Age: 42

Sex: Female

Race: Pacific Islander

Occupation: Emergency Management Specialist

Alanna works for a consulting firm that contracts with agencies all around the world to conduct analyses and recommend protocols for emergency situations. Her department's focus is transportation. They cover everything from shipping and disruptions in the fuel supply chain to potential road closures and stalled public transportation. Even though she spends her days thinking about disasters, Alanna finds her work fascinating.

Alanna's summer job in college was working as an adventure guide. The required training in wilderness first aid. The company she worked for had an excellent safety so she never had to open her first aid kit for a client. The training did pique her interest in emergency services. When she got back to school found out that could change her major from marketing to emergency management. She was easily able to find a job after graduation.

Alanna does not have any major or chronic health problems. When she was working as an adventure guide, she contracted dengue fever. She was very sick for a few days, but recovered quickly. Other than having all four of her wisdom teeth extracted when she was 18, Alanna has never had surgery. She works out at the gym a couple days a week and generally tries to a healthy diet.

Alanna's father is a colon cancer survivor. To help his recovery her mother put her father on a strict diet. He frequently texts Alanna and her brother with pleas to "stop by and bring some decent food." Her mother takes medication for hypertension. Alanna's maternal grandmother is 96 and living on her own in the same house where she raised her family. Alanna wants to live a long life like her grandmother.

The gym where Alanna works out just hired a new Pilates instructor. Alana signed up for a class. She has done Pilates before and found it to be a very relaxing work out.

Case Notes

Sam

Age: 65

Sex: Male

Race: Black

Occupation: Actor

Sam is a sought-after character actor. He is best known for tough, smart, and capable roles. He has played cowboys, police officers, security guards, thugs, and gangsters. People often tell him that he looks familiar, but they cannot figure out why until he mentions a film or television show. Then they recognized him immediately from one of his roles. He became an actor because he enjoys the work, not because he wanted to be famous. Still, it is fun when people recognize him.

Sam works very hard to stay fit for his work. He works out every day, sometimes twice a day. When he is home, he lifts weights at the gym, alternating days for different muscles. He uses the elliptical machine or a stationary bicycle for a half hour of cardio every day. He also takes an Aikido class a few times per week. For Sam, going to the gym or Aikido class is social, so it is good for both mind and body.

Sometimes Sam has delayed onset muscle soreness after intense workouts. To alleviate discomfort, he stretches or ices his muscles. Being sore is necessary for him to stay in shape.

Sam's father was a high school basketball coach. He preached conditioning for his players. Sam played for him all four years and won a scholarship to college. Many of Sam's teammates in college sustained knee injuries but not Sam. He made it through high school and college basketball without any major injuries. He credits his commitment to working out in the weight room and stretching like his father taught him with keeping him injury-free.

Sam's father died at age 77 from prostate cancer. His mother died when she was 74 from lung cancer. None of his grandparents lived past age 70. Sam is committed to living a long healthy life.

On one of his last jobs one of the featured actresses brought along a piece of Pilates equipment. The design was unusual and Sam was intrigued. Now he is interested in trying Pilates.

Case Notes

Constanza

Age: 49

Sex: Female

Race: White

Occupation: Social Worker

Constanza is a program manager at a nonprofit. The organization is dedicated to the well-being of refugees. Constanza's program coordinates with community partners to furnish homes for families settling into the community. She organizes donations of furniture, toys, clothing, and personal-care items to create a comfortable space for new arrivals. Many of the refugees served by the program have fled violence and political strife. It is difficult for Constanza to think about what they have experienced. but she takes pride in knowing her work is making a positive difference in their lives.

Stress management is important for Constanza. Not only because of her work, but also because she has hypertension. She takes medication and received an activity tracker through a wellness program. Her goal is to take 10,000 steps every day. Constanza always exceeds her goal on days she goes work. She listens to music every night before going to bed. It helps her unwind and clear her head. On weekends Constanza tends to a small herb garden on her patio. She finds gardening to be a meditative activity. It is a good stress reliever.

Heart disease runs in Constanza's family. Her parents, brother, and two sisters all suffer from hypertension. Constanza knows lifestyle modification can improve her health. She tries to eat a healthy diet, but many days she grabs fast food for lunch between meetings with store managers and scouting trips to thrift shops.

Constanza has a milestone birthday coming up. She is trying to get inspired to be healthier in her next decade. A few years ago she took a Pilates class at a resort when she was on vacation. It was fun and challenging. Constanza decided to sing up for a small group Pilates class. If she likes it then she plans to make it part of her regular wellness routine.

Case Notes

William

Age: 37

Sex: Male

Race: Alaska Native

Occupation: Tour Guide

William gives wildlife tours. He leads small groups of guests through backcountry to see wild animals in their natural habitat. Depending upon the season and itinerary, they travel by Jeep, bus, or boat. William's job is to ensure the safety of guests and also to make sure they have adequate time at points of interest. For most guests, the trip is a once-in-a-lifetime experience.

Typical tour staff includes two guides and a porter. For overnight trips there are additional porters and a chef. William has worked with some of the same staff since he started at the company over a decade ago. They have learned that working together helps everything run smoothly.

William has an excellent guest safety record, but he has sustained a few injuries over the years. He broke his leg skiing and fractured his nose when he got hit with a paddle on a rafting trip. For him, that is all in a day's work.

Staying healthy is important for William's work and well-being. Because his work is very physical, when he feels sore, tired, or run down it can be difficult to run a tour. It can potentially be dangerous. If a guest needs help or gets into trouble, William needs to spring into action. He needs to be physically and mentally present on every tour.

William is the youngest of two. His father is a physician and his mother is an artist. William's brother always wanted to be a physician, but William was drawn to the wilderness. William earned a degree in occupational safety and briefly worked in the fuel industry before joining the tour company. He loves being outdoors and cannot imagine working at any other job.

As he has gotten older, William has definitely noticed changes in his body. He is not as strong or flexible as he was when he was younger. He recognizes that he needs make a plan to stay fit and healthy. A client on a recent tour owned a Pilates studio. William thought it sounded very interesting and wants to find a class.

Case Notes

Chloe

Age: 27

Sex: Female

Race: Black

Occupation: Painter

Chloe started working for her father's painting business during the summer when she was in high school. He wanted her to learn a responsibility and a trade. She fit right in with the crew and helped the business grow. Chloe's father was a veteran and he was her role model. She felt it was important to serve and she was determined to succeed in business. When she graduated from high school, Chloe enlisted in the Army National Guard. After basic training she joined the painting business full-time.

Chloe's grandmother came to live with them when Chloe was 12, after her mother died from breast cancer. Her grandmother took care of the housework, packed Chloe's lunch, and made sure Chloe did her homework. She helped Chloe and her dad heal. Chloe became very close to her grandmother.

When Chloe started complaining of abdominal pain, her grandmother thought it was psychosomatic. She let Chloe take time off school, gave her a hot water bottle and made her tea. As the pain persisted, she began to worry, so she took Chloe to the community clinic. After that first appointment it took a long time and a lot of visits to the clinic to get an accurate diagnosis of endometriosis. Once she was diagnosed, Chloe underwent treatment and her pain got better.

Other than endometriosis, Chloe does not have any major health problems. She regularly runs and does strength training to stay fit for her work in the Army National Guard. Sometimes she gets sore from her workouts. Occasionally her neck and shoulders are sore after work.

Lately Chloe has been busier than usual. Several of her friends are getting married next year. Chloe will be a bridesmaid at two of their weddings

One of the brides-to-be is determined to get in shape with Pilates. She convinced Chloe to join her at a small group apparatus class. Chloe hopes it won't make her neck worse.

Case Notes

Maria

Age: 53

Sex: Female

Race: White

Occupation: Classroom Aide

Maria is a mother of four and grandmother of two. She loves children and started working as a classroom aide twelve years ago helping children with special needs. Because she is bilingual, Maria also works as a translator at the school. Maria likes making a difference in the lives of her students and their families. Her dedication and hard work has earned her respect from the teachers, staff, and parents.

At the end of the day Maria's feet are often swollen. Her shoes are so tight it hurts her feet. She elevates her legs after dinner and sometimes uses a topical analgesic to relieve the discomfort. The swelling and discomfort seems to have gotten worse over the years.

Maria is prediabetic. She has been overweight since she had her first child. She likes to cook and has never really exercised. During her fourth pregnancy, Maria had preeclampsia. Her obstetrician told her that would increase the risk of developing hypertension. She now takes a low dose aspirin every day and regularly monitors her blood pressure.

Maria's father was a factory worker who died of liver cancer. Her mother had heart disease. Maria's husband was recently diagnosed with Type 2 diabetes. Maria's mother-in-law had diabetes and had to have her leg amputated. Maria and her husband want him to avoid a similar fate. They know they will have to make lifestyle changes. They have signed up for a diabetes prevention program offered at the local community center.

Maria and her husband know they need to exercise. Her husband and one of his friends joined a gym. They started working out together three days a week. Thinks the gym is intimidating. One of the staff at school told her about a Pilates class at the community center. She said they exercise a lot of the time while lying down. Maria thinks that sounds kind of weird but she is going to try a class on the weekend.

Case Notes

Taima

Age: 42

Sex: Male

Race: American Indian

Occupation: Health Educator

Taima is committed to wellness. He studied health promotion in college and earned certifications as a health educator and a personal trainer. For a number of years, Taima worked at a corporate fitness facility. He started out as a fitness trainer was promoted to assistant manager. Taima got married and had two children. He and his wife worked hard to stay healthy.

One of Taima's cousins told him that the community clinic received a grant for health promotion and was hiring. Taima applied for a position as a health educator and was offered a job. Taima was excited for the opportunity to give back to the community. He works with individual clients and runs support groups on lifestyle modification. Taima finds his work very rewarding.

Many of his clients have help problems related to stress and health behaviors. Taima and the program director created "stress management menu" journaling, breathing exercises, gentle movement, listening to music, and other relaxing activities. He teaches his clients to select one item from the menu every day to give themselves a relaxation break. Taima tries to make sure that he regularly uses a strategy on his "menu" to help cope with stress.

Taima's parents, his sister, and two brothers all have some type of chronic health problem: diabetes, asthma, and/or hypertension. Being overweight seems to run in the family. These are the things that sparked Taima's interest in wellness and health promotion.

A new physical therapist at the community clinic is also a certified Pilates teacher. She is going to offer a group class on the weekends. Taima is going to try the class so he can learn about Pilates and possibly recommend it to his clients in the lifestyle modification program.

Case Notes

Agatha

Age: 73

Sex: Female

Race: White

Occupation: Retired Nurse

Agatha is busier in retirement than she ever thought possible. She works part-time at a department store and volunteers as a tutor in an after-school program. She sings in church choir and hosts a family dinner at her house most Sundays.

Agatha worked for over forty years as a post-anesthesia care unit nurse at a regional hospital. After her children were grown, she traveled on an annual medical mission with an organization that provided surgical care in remote areas. For Agatha, the missions were a balance between service and adventure.

Agatha's feet have always bothered her. They were often swollen after a shift at the hospital. She always had to choose her shoes carefully for her shift at the hospital and must do the same at the department store to accommodate the inevitable swelling and discomfort.

Agatha takes medication for hypertension and high cholesterol. She is a little overweight and has long struggled to lose weight. When the weather is nice, Agatha meets a neighbor for a morning walk. Agatha's feet are rarely swollen after she goes walking.

Other than her swollen feet, Agatha has had few health problems. One winter, she fell on the ice and broke her wrist.

She had cataract surgery when she was in her early fifties. Agatha had a terrible time with night sweats during menopause.

Agatha's mother died a few years ago at age 96 from pneumonia. Her father died of heart disease when he was 68. Agatha's son and daughter both have hypertension.

One of Agatha's friends from the department store started taking Pilates class. She got a pass for a free class and invited Agatha to join her. Agatha wonders if it will bother her feet or her wrist.

Case Notes

Neena

Age: 39

Sex: Female

Race: Asian

Occupation: Physician

Neena is an endocrinologist. She works at an urban academic health center and is becoming recognized for her work with rare diseases. Many of her patients are complex cases with unusual or persistent symptoms. They often travel from far away for a consultation. Neena is fortunate to be able to spend time with the patients during these consultations. Many of her colleagues only see patients for very short appointments. For Neena learning the patient's stories and digging into their backgrounds can help identify potentially relevant tests and referrals for treatments.

Between her consultations with patients and teaching medical students, Neena's days are very full. Her neck and upper back are usually stiff by the time she leaves work. Neena often puts a heat wrap on her neck when she gets home from work. Sometimes chair massages are offered at work. When she can get a massage her neck feels better for a day or two.

Neena has three young children. They spend time after school at her mother-in-law's house. By the time Neena or her husband pick them up, they have had snacks and their homework is finished. This helps evenings run smoothly for her family. But being a mom is a lot of work.

Both of Neena's parents have diabetes, as did both of her grandmothers. That is what inspired her interest in endocrinology. Neena wants to avoid the same fate. She watches what she eats and tries to take 10,000 steps every day. She does not have time to go to a gym but she knows she needs to exercise.

One of the nurses in Neena's department started taking a lunch time Pilates class at a studio not far from work. She has been raving about the class and how good it makes her feel. The nurse is trying to get everyone to join her to help the instructor fill the class so they can make a lunchtime series permanent on the studio schedule.

Case Notes

Dion

Age: 63

Sex: Male

Race: Black

Occupation: Marketing Executive

Dion works for a large cosmetics company in the perfume division. His group specializes in developing and marketing celebrity-branded fragrances. Dion does a lot of research into competitive brands, possible scents, and packaging and branding. Dion's days are full of meetings within the company and with potential distribution outlets. He travels extensively.

Dion is a former professional football player. He was drafted right out of college and played professionally for three years until he was sidelined by a knee injury. Dion leveraged his degree in business and connections in the players association to get a job in marketing at a personal care products company. He worked his way up the corporate ladder. The cosmetics company recruited him specifically to expand their business. Dion has done well and earned some nice bonuses. Dion is proud of the career he built in marketing.

His injury—a torn ACL, MCL, and meniscus—is common in football. He had surgery and went through physical therapy, but his leg never returned to full function. That was why he had to stop playing football. Every so often his knee still acts up. He manages the problem with his own protocol of ice, heat, and stretches to help it feel better.

Other than the knee problem, Dion is pretty healthy for his age. His only other issue is occasional back pain. He works out three times a week at the gym when he is home and does calisthenics when he is traveling. He tries to go to group cycling class twice a week. His blood pressure is a little elevated, so he takes a low dose aspirin every day.

Dion still follows news about his old professional team. In a recent newsletter they mentioned having the players do Pilates. Dion wonders if it might help his back and do anything his knee.

Case Notes

Isoke

Age: 21

Sex: Female

Race: Black

Occupation: Student

Isoke is a communications major in her final term of college. She is looking for a job in media or public relations. Isoke has had a few interviews, but has not yet received a job offer. She is getting stressed, especially because several of her sorority sisters have already landed jobs. Isoke is trying to stay positive, but she is feeling increasingly run-down. Fatigue is something Isoke has to carefully monitor because she has sickle cell disease. Fatigue and exertion can trigger widespread pain, so Isoke has learned to be strict with herself to get adequate rest. She thinks the fatigue is really just stress and anxiety.

Isoke is an only child. She was raised by her mother who worked very hard to create a regimen to help manage her symptoms. This included gentle exercise every day, a healthy diet, and relaxation time before bed to help her get to sleep at night. In elementary school, Isoke was enrolled in a special gym class since she had to be careful about overexertion. In high school she was exempt from gym class. That was partly why her mother had her do gentle exercises at home every day.

Isoke's uncle and grandmother also had sickle cell disease and they had many complications. Isoke saw firsthand how awful the pain and fatigue could be. She is thankful that her mother helped her develop a self-care routine.

Isoke takes medication and supplements every day and is careful about her diet. Three or four days a week, she does a low-intensity cardio workout at the campus fitness center. Isoke has developed a self-care routine that she plans to continue when she starts working. But first, she needs to land a job.

Several of Isoke's sorority sisters have started taking Pilates at a studio near campus. They describe it is gentle exercise. Isoke is interested to see if it might be something that she can tolerate.

Case Notes

Nathan

Age: 29

Sex: Male

Race: Multiracial

Occupation: Physical Therapy Assistant

Nathan works at a large rehabilitation facility. He got interested in physical therapy as a high school student. Nathan injured his ankle playing basketball and did a few rounds of rehabilitation. He quizzed the staff about career possibilities. Nathan was able to get his degree as physical therapy assistant and play on the basketball team at the community college. Nathan loves his work and takes pride in his ability to connect with patients.

Occasionally, Nathan's ankle bothers him. It is a combination of pain, weakness, and functional limitation. Sometimes when he is walking downstairs, his ankle freezes and he has to grab the handrail. Multiple doctor visits, imaging tests, and assessments have not identified any structural causes.

Nathan works out four or five days a week, alternating cardio and strength training. He also does balance training for his ankle. He plays an occasional pick-up game with friends and is a volunteer coach for a youth basketball league.

Nathan's father was also a basketball player in high school. Now, he has hypertension and Type 2 diabetes. He has struggled with his weight for years. Nathan's mother is overweight and has osteoarthritis in her knee. She is scheduled for knee replacement surgery. Nathan sees patients who are struggling to rehabilitate from conditions caused by their lifestyle. He wants his parents to be healthy. He is worried about them.

A few of the physical therapists and exercise physiologists at work are certified Pilates teachers. Nathan has watched them do some exercises with their patients. It looked really interesting so Nathan is now interested in trying Pilates.

Case Notes

Guadalupe

Age: 31

Sex: Female

Race: White

Occupation: Veterinary Technician

Guadalupe started running when she was 23. She made a resolution to get in shape and wanted to spend time outdoors. She followed a walk-to-run program for beginning runners. Within a few months she was logging 15 miles per week. Guadalupe joined a running club and started doing group runs on the weekends. She entered a few road races for fun and set a goal to run a half marathon. Guadalupe enjoyed the longer distances. She regularly runs 40 miles per week. Her running evolved into a program to help mind and body. It helps her stay fit and manage stress.

Guadalupe's calf muscles get tight. She has heard from other runners that stress fractures are common, and she wants to avoid that fate. She stretches and uses a massage stick after she runs.

Guadalupe's family owns a restaurant. Her father was diagnosed with Type 2 diabetes when Guadalupe was 23; that was her inspiration to get in shape. Both of her parents now have diabetes. As restaurateurs, it was difficult to change their diet. Guadalupe finally convinced them to go walking in the mornings before work. Guadalupe's maternal grandmother also has diabetes. She suffers from debilitating neuropathy in her feet and uses a walker to get around.

Guadalupe is determined to stay fit and healthy. She is glad to have made friends in the running club. The support from other runners helps inspire her to get out of bed and run before work. She loves seeing everyone races on the weekends.

Several members of her running group joined a new Pilates studio. The private sessions are too expensive for Guadalupe's budget. The small group sessions and mat classes are a more formal option. Guadalupe is going to sign up for an introductory series to see if Pilates can help her stay healthy.

Case Notes

Iosefa

Age: 56

Sex: Male

Race: Pacific Islander

Occupation: Clinical Trial Manager

Iosefa works for an international contract research organization. He manages one arm of a large clinical drug trial. Much of his work involves forms and budgets. Iosefa's days are filled with preparing, reviewing, or auditing documents, along with meetings and conference calls. He has been working in clinical research for a long time. The order and organization required by his job suits his nature.

Iosefa was diagnosed with HIV when he was 42 years old. He takes antiretroviral medication and supplements. Sometimes he feels nauseated (a common medication side effect) and he often has trouble sleeping and was diagnosed with insomnia . Thankfully, he works from home and has a flexible schedule, so he can nap during the day when he is fatigued.

When Iosefa was first diagnosed with HIV, he was angry but not entirely surprised. He quickly became determined to do all he could to promote his own health. Complying with treatment was more difficult than he anticipated, so Iosefa started a medication log. In time, he expanded it to an overall health journal. He logs his daily activity, foods eaten, and stress level in addition to medication. Iosefa spent years working with clinical health data. Creating his own personal dataset has been very interesting.

A side effect of Iosefa's current medication is that it can lead to heart disease. Both of Iosefa's parents had heart disease and died before they were 70. He views this as increased risk that he could develop heart disease. Insomnia is another side effect of his medication, which might account for his difficulty sleeping but it also could be stress. He knows that stress can be problematic for HIV patients, so he wants to take a more comprehensive approach to stress management. Iosefa read an article about Pilates. It described gentle exercise that was good for fitness and stress reduction. Iosefa immediately signed up for a group class.

Case Notes

Carol

Age: 43

Sex: Female

Race: Black

Occupation: Spa Manager

Carol manages a luxury day spa. They are known for their decadent body treatments and Moroccan-inspired design. Guests can select a chocolate wrap, coconut scrub, mojito pedicure, or other unique service in addition to a massage or facial. They change the special body treatments based upon the season and upcoming holidays. Carol loves the creative aspect of the spa menu and making subtle changes to the products and decor to maintain a luxurious atmosphere.

Carol's first job was at a cosmetic, body care, and fragrance retail store. She learned a lot about skincare and about retail. Carol thought about pursuing cosmetology training, but instead earned a certificate in hospitality and spa management. She worked at a few day spas before landing her current position.

Carol and her staff work hard to ensure that each guest feels like a VIP. Carol has learned ways to deal with difficult guests, so her staff looks to her to diffuse difficult situations. Carol learned a lot about difficult clients from her training and also from her partner. They met when her (now) partner catered a bridal shower that Carol attended. The two of them bonded over discussions about challenges serving high-end clientele. They went on their first date a week later and have been together ever since. Sometimes their work schedules are difficult to align, but they managed to make time for each other.

Carol has developed some chronic problems with her right arm. She was diagnosed with tennis elbow, but Carol does not play tennis. Her doctor suspects it is related to her computer use at work. When Carol has discomfort, she uses a hot towel or topical analgesic. At home, she uses a microwaveable heat pack.

Carol and her partner made a resolution to get fit. They signed up for a small group Pilates class to spend time together and exercise.

Case Notes

Nihal

Age: 33

Sex: Male

Race: Asian

Occupation: Data Analyst

Nihal is a self-professed computer nerd. When he was growing up, his parents made him finish his homework before he could play computer games. Otherwise his homework would never get done. Nihal learned to start doing his homework on the school bus so he could finish it faster and get to his computer for gaming.

Nihal went to a computer camp every summer that was held at a local university. The campers would spend the mornings playing outdoor games and the afternoons in the computer lab building apps and websites. Every morning, Nihal would struggle through the games looking forward to the computer lab. What he liked most at camp was spending time with other kids that had the same love of computers.

Nihal went to college and earned a degree in computer science. Before he graduated he was hired by a tech startup. Ever since he has spent his day right where he wanted to be: at the computer. The startup is doing well. His office is casual and has an open floor plan. Some of the employees bring their dogs to work. He likes his colleagues, the dogs, and the laid back environment

Nihal sometimes suffers from neck and upper back pain. He tries to stretch or use a heat wrap. Nihal has never sustained any neck injuries. No one in his family suffers from neck problems or neurological conditions. Nihal is fairly certain that his neck problems are related to work because he spends long hours there. He does go to group cycling class three or four times a week and occasionally goes for long bike rides with a friend on the weekends.

Someone posted a flyer in the break room for a new Pilates studio in the building. It mentions something about back pain. Nihal is curious to try and see if it might be good for neck pain too.

Case Notes

Magdalena

Age: 69

Sex: Female

Race: White

Occupation: Store Owner

Magdalena owns a boutique. She stocks an eclectic array of gifts and home décor items. From candles to costume jewelry, scarves, and figurines, her store is the place to go for anyone looking for a special and unusual gift. Magdelena's boutique has been a fixture in town for nearly 25 years.

Magdalena has suffered from back pain for decades. Lately it has become more persistent. It has been difficult for her to get through a whole day at work without sitting to take a break. When she first opened the boutique she was so busy she rarely sat down. Now her back bothers her so much, she spends most of her time in the back office while her staff manages the floor.

Magdalena has struggled with her weight since she had her first baby. She tried every diet imaginable and seemed to only gain weight with every diet she tried. She has little interest in exercise because she does not like to sweat. Once, when her back pain was very bad, she went to the doctor. After several tests did not find anything wrong, she was referred to physical therapy. Magdalena did not enjoy the physical therapy sessions, but she felt better afterwards. Some of the exercises were very simple. Recently Magdalena close the back office door and tried a few of them. She was surprised it helped her back feel better.

Magdalena's father had kidney disease, so he often had back pain. He had to follow a very restricted diet and ended up on dialysis when he was older. Magdalena's grandmother died from kidney disease. Magdalena tries not to think about it happening to her too.

Other than her weight and the back pain, Magdalena does not have any health problems. She knows if she can get the back pain under control it will improve her quality of life. The movement studio down the street started offering Pilates mat classes. Magdalena has resolved to try a class.

Case Notes

Gavin

Age: 47

Sex: Male

Race: Black

Occupation: Insurance Agent

Gavin started working in financial services after he graduated from college. A friend of his uncle's recommended Gavin for a corporate training program in a large city. Gavin enjoyed city life. He lived in a tiny apartment and went to clubs, restaurants, and the theatre. When Gavin's mother was diagnosed with breast cancer, he moved back home to be near her. Gavin found a job selling insurance, got married, and started a family. He has settled into life in the small town where he grew up.

Gavin strained groin muscle again. It has been a persistent problem since high school. He strained his hip in high school during marching band practice. Every so often it flares up again, the exact same pain he had with the first injury. All through school Gavin was in marching band. He played the trombone from middle school through college. Gavin's closest friends were from band. They still keep in touch and have reunions.

Gavin's father has hypertension and high cholesterol. He is an elementary school principal. Their mother worked part-time at a nursing home. Gavin and his sister learned at a young age to keep up with their schoolwork and get their chores done. When their mother injured her back at work, Gavin and his sister took care of the housework until she got better. They did the same when she was undergoing cancer treatment. His mother is now cancer free but her back still bothers her.

This time Gavin's groin muscle problem was aggravated when he was teaching his son to throw a football. He did not warm up before they went into the yard. Gavin learned about warm-ups in marching band. Once this strain is healed, he is resolved to always warm up before playing. Right now he just needs to stretch out his muscles to make the pain and tightness go away. His wife suggested he take a class with her Pilates teacher.

Case Notes

Alain

Age: 38

Sex: Male

Race: White

Occupation: Translator

Alain is fluent in five languages. His father was a foreign service officer. By the time he graduated high school, Alain had lived on three continents. His family always tried to get to know the language, customs, and food in every region where they lived. Nearly place that he lived and every school he attended had a soccer team or club. Alain made many friends playing soccer.

Becoming a translator was an easy decision for Alain. He had a natural affinity for languages. His family spoke English and French at home. Alain studied Spanish, German, and Russian in school. He went to work for an nongovernment organization specializing in international issues related to science and help. Alain spends most of his time preparing written translations, but he also does live translations for large meetings. His work always requires serious concentration.

Alain's neck bothers him. The problem is always on the left side. The pattern is the same. He feels a shooting pain from his neck to his shoulder and his neck is stiff. It is very difficult to turn his head.

Alain injured his neck in a surfing accident when he was 17. It was a minor injury, but it required that he wear a neck brace for a few months. He couldn't play soccer for a while but eventually got back on the field. Some persistent stiffness and discomfort started a few years later when he was working on his college thesis when he spent long hours in the library with his laptop. Usually the stiffness went away after he stretched. In recent years, getting rid of the discomfort has required more effort. He has had more MRIs than he can count. None have revealed a structural cause related to his symptoms.

Alain is looking to update his self-care plan. He knows he needs to exercise and take care of his neck. A few of his friends from soccer started taking Pilates. Alain is curious to see what it is all about.

Case Notes

Index

About the Author

Virginia S. Cowen, PhD is a researcher, writer, and educator with over 20 years' experience in health, fitness and wellness. She has been a member of the faculty at Rutgers University, University of Medicine and Dentistry of New Jersey, and Queensborough Community College. Dr. Cowen earned her PhD in curriculum and instruction with a concentration in exercise and wellness from Arizona State University. She is a Google Certified Educator Level 1 and Level 2. She has served on the research committee for the Pilates Method Alliance. She is a Nationally Certified Pilates Teacher, a licensed massage therapist, and holds certifications as a yoga teacher, strength and conditioning specialist, and personal trainer.

Other Books by Virginia S. Cowen, PhD

Hands Off! 70 Active Learning Strategies for Pilates Teacher Training —Pennate Press

Beyond Lectures: Engaging Distance Learning for Pilates Teacher Training —Pennate Press

Hands Off! 70 Active Learning Strategies for Exercise Science and Personal Training —Pennate Press

Beyond Lectures: Engaging Distance Learning for Exercise Science and Personal Training —Pennate Press

101 Cases for Study in Exercise Science and Personal Training —Pennate Press

Hands Off! 70 Active Learning Strategies for Massage and Bodywork Education —Pennate Press

Beyond Lectures: Engaging Distance Learning for Massage and Bodywork Education —Pennate Press

101 Cases for Study in Massage and Bodywork Education —Pennate Press

Hands Off! 70 Active Learning Strategies for Yoga Teacher Training —Pennate Press

101 Cases for Study in Yoga Teacher Training —Pennate Press

Pathophysiology for Massage Therapists: A Functional Approach —F.A. Davis

Therapeutic Massage and Bodywork for Autism Spectrum Disorders: A Guide for Parents and Caregivers —Singing Dragon Books